WORLD HEALTH ORGANIZATION
MONOGRAPH SERIES
No. 1

PSYCHIATRIC ASPECTS OF
JUVENILE DELINQUENCY

PSYCHIATRIC ASPECTS
OF
JUVENILE DELINQUENCY

A study prepared on behalf of the World Health Organization
as a contribution to the United Nations programme for the
prevention of crime and treatment of offenders

LUCIEN BOVET, M.D.

*Médecin-chef de l'Office médico-pédagogique rattaché au
Département de Justice et Police de l'Etat de Vaud, Lausanne, Switzerland
Consultant in Mental Health, World Health Organization*

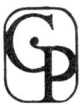

GREENWOOD PRESS, PUBLISHERS
WESTPORT, CONNECTICUT

BOWLING GREEN STATE UNIVERSITY LIBRARY

Originally published in 1951
by World Health Organization

Reprinted from a copy in the collections
of the Brooklyn Public Library

First Greenwood Reprinting 1970

SBN 8371-3019-0

PRINTED IN UNITED STATES OF AMERICA

CONTENTS

		Page
1.	General considerations on juvenile delinquency	7
1.1	Concept of juvenile delinquency	8
1.2	Present knowledge	10
2	Etiology of juvenile delinquency	12
2.1	General observations on social adaptation in the normal child	12
2.2	Sociological factors	18
2.3	Somatic and constitutional factors	21
2.4	Disturbances in the psychological development of the personality	31
2.5	Secondary community influences: cinema, radio, the press, alcoholism	37
2.6	Conclusions — Psychological common denominator of criminal factors	41
3	Prevention of juvenile delinquency	43
3.1	General observations: aims and functions of prophylaxis	43
3.2	Sociological factors	48
3.3	Somatic and constitutional factors	50
3.4	Disturbances in the psychological development of the personality	53
3.5	Secondary community influences: cinema, radio, the press, alcoholism	58
3.6	Conclusions	59
4	Treatment of juvenile delinquency	62
4.1	"Primum non nocere"	62
4.2	Clinical examination	63
4.3	Outpatient treatment	66
4.4	Residential treatment	67
4.5	Delinquents on licence	74
4.6	After-care	75
4.7	Training of staff	76
4.8	Conclusions	77
Summary and general conclusions		79
Bibliography		87

CHAPTER 1

GENERAL CONSIDERATIONS ON JUVENILE DELINQUENCY

On 13 August 1948 the Economic and Social Council of the United Nations recommended that the Secretary-General convene a committee of experts to advise the Secretary-General and the Social Commission on the ways and means of formulating a suitable programme for :

"(a) The study on an international basis of the prevention of crime and the treatment of offenders ; and

(b) International action in this field."[129]

At the beginning of August 1949 this committee of experts met at Lake Success and agreed that juvenile delinquency in all its aspects was of particular importance and its study should be given priority.

Since the study of juvenile delinquency includes important medical and psychiatric problems, the committee further advised that WHO in particular should be asked to participate. This suggestion was accepted by the Secretary-General of the United Nations. The report, therefore, on the first session of the Expert Committee on Mental Health, held in Geneva at the end of August 1949, contains the following paragraph (page 27) : [137]

" The committee welcomed the request by the United Nations for the contribution by WHO to their study of a memorandum on the psychiatric aspects of juvenile delinquency. It recommends that WHO should appoint a short-term consultant ... to prepare a concise but comprehensive summary of existing psychiatric views on this matter."

The Chief of the Mental Health Section of WHO, in a letter to a member of the committee, described the consultant's task in the following terms :

" It is planned to appoint a short-term specialist adviser on a temporary contract, to prepare a memorandum for UN on the psychiatric aspects of the etiology, prevention, and treatment of juvenile delinquency. We would like this memorandum to be a general review of the most widely accepted opinions in this field today, and to draw attention to the work of those institutes and individuals, which should be known to all criminologists. Naturally, it is not intended that this review should be of a strictly scientific nature, but rather a broad picture for the intelligent reader, without psychiatric training."

To accomplish this task and with these terms of reference, the Director-General of WHO appointed the present writer, and work was started in December 1949. The main part of my work, preparatory to writing this report, consisted of a tour of several European countries and America, during which I had the privilege of consulting over 150 specialists of all kinds in juvenile delinquency, and of visiting 60 institutes of diverse nature.

After much thought, and after discussion with the Chief of the Mental Health Section of WHO, and the Deputy Director of the Social Activities Division of UN, it was decided that a personal synthesis would best serve the desired purpose rather than an objective enumeration of current views and opinions, which might prove tedious to read and be of doubtful value. I do not wish to conceal the subjective nature of this report, but I hope thereby to paint a more vivid picture, inspired by the numerous impressions of my travels. However personal this report may be, it nevertheless reflects the varying opinions and tendencies in Europe and the USA today. Since I was limited for time, I could not attempt a complete and worldwide survey of psychiatric opinion on juvenile delinquency. I therefore had to resort to sampling ideas, taking those I thought more or less typical, though not always the most outstanding, or necessarily the only valuable ones. Material difficulties influenced my choice of countries visited and people consulted, rather than any formal appraisal of merit. Indeed, the extent of the omissions in my list of sources readily shows that the absence of any particular reference should in no way be taken as a derogatory judgement thereof.

1.1 Concept of Juvenile Delinquency

To the lawyer, the concept of juvenile delinquency is clear-cut and is given a precise definition in law. As Rubin [107] tersely remarks: "juvenile delinquency is what the law says it is".

My first point is that, in contrast to this precise legal concept, neither psychiatry nor psychology can offer any such unequivocal formulation. Delinquency is not the name of an illness, nor is there one simple specific psychological category for all delinquents, and for them alone. Yet still today, doctors, magistrates, and teachers seem to be dominated, though often almost unconsciously, by a belief in a specific psycho-biological delinquent type. In this connexion, the following facts should be borne in mind. In the first place, the legal definition of juvenile delinquency varies from one country to another. Thus, in many European countries, a minor is legally considered a delinquent only if his breach of the penal code is an offence for the whole population. On the other hand, in other countries, particularly in the USA, the charges on which a minor appears before a court cover a wide range of behaviour: truancy from school, consistent disobedience to parents, consumption of alcohol, smoking in public (to give but a few examples), are all considered juvenile offences. But even if a nation's laws were to be based on psychological considerations, owing to the intrinsic nature of a law, they could not be applied to every individual with anything like the degree of subtlety a psychologist would require. The law must contain an arbitrary element. This point is well illustrated by the problem of the maximum and minimum ages at which a particular procedure or measure is to be applied. Pearce [89] gives the following excellent example: according to English law, a boy is not considered capable of having sexual relations before his 14th birthday, so that a juvenile court was powerless to return a verdict other than " not guilty " in the case of a boy, aged $13^{1}/_{2}$, who had raped a small girl, thereby causing her death. In addition, the way the police enforce the law, whether more or less strictly, introduces from the psychologist's point of view a further arbitrary element into the concept of juvenile delinquency. A country with an efficient police-force will have a higher delinquency-rate than a country where the police are slack. It is true that, in any country, the decision on whether to refer a boy to a juvenile court may often depend on the social position and influence of his parents. Finally, the severity with which an offence is viewed may vary a great deal, not only from one country to another, but also from one judge to another, thereby introducing a further psychologically false factor into the concept of juvenile delinquency.

These examples alone prove that juvenile delinquents do not fall into one simple homogeneous psychiatric or psychological category. As I shall show later, particularly in the chapter on etiological factors, the distinction between delinquents and non-delinquents, especially when applied to minors, is not only arbitrary but is also often based on factors which have quantitative, rather than specific qualitative, differences. In other words, certain personal or social factors, in themselves neither pathological nor specific, will by their degree of intensity cause an individual to be given the legal classification of delinquent, whilst psychologically there is little if anything to distinguish him from others who have escaped legal sanctions.

It would, of course, be absurd to deny the correlation between delinquency and psychological or psychiatric facts. Indeed the very aim of this report is to point out these correlations and to draw the necessary practical conclusions. While according to the lawyer and, to a certain extent, to the sociologist and the teacher, juvenile delinquents form a well-defined group, according to the psychologist and psychiatrist delinquency is but one of the many aspects of that elusive concept, social maladjustment. The psychologist observes that within a society, or even within a group, there are some individuals who can obey and follow those rules and taboos most commonly accepted in that group or society, whilst for others this is impossible. The latter do not form a psychologically homogeneous group, but psychology can help explain their behaviour, and, although the majority of juvenile delinquents are found among them, not all are delinquent. Furthermore, not all delinquents are maladjusted. That the majority of a nation or society accepts certain rules and taboos does not imply that all the groups in that nation or society will equally accept them. Similarly, the laws of a nation or a government are not recognized by all as final.

One can imagine, for example, an individual driven by a strong religious conscience breaking the law and thereby coming into conflict with society, without his being labelled as " maladjusted ". More frequently still, delinquent behaviour can be adaptive, meeting the special circumstances in which a group finds itself, although such behaviour clashes with the generally accepted laws of the society to which the group belongs. This is particularly true in certain quarters of many big towns, and in exceptional times, such as during wars and revolutions.

In one respect however, the group of juvenile delinquents appears homogeneous to the psychiatrist. Once a juvenile delinquent, whatever his make-up, has been classified as such and has been subjected to various measures, secondary psychological reactions occur, unrelated to the origins of his delinquent behaviour but common to all who share his fate. On the other hand, public opinion and all " right-minded " people, because he has been labelled delinquent, take up special attitudes towards him, regardless of the individual features of his case.[102] The psychiatric and psychological study of both sides' reactions is essential if juvenile delinquents are to be effectively dealt with, or if the unpleasant consequences which society's treatment of the juvenile delinquent entails are to be modified.

While this report is written from a psychiatric, and thereby to a certain extent from a psychological, point of view, there are many other aspects of juvenile delinquency, legal, sociological, educational, and administrative. At times the demands of the psychiatrist will clash with those of other specialists. When, therefore, each of the different specialists has thought out his side of the problem and has put forward the requirements implied by his particular approach (this report being an example of a psychiatric formulation of the problem), all the specialists, their individual positions thus concisely stated and defined, should meet, and, exploring differences in point of view and conclusions, should make an overall and common synthesis. Reports such as this are hence but the initial steps in the creation of a " juvenile criminology " long wished for by Professor Heuyer, among many others.

This report, in dealing with the psychiatric approach to juvenile delinquency, must at times encroach on the spheres of interest of other workers whether legal, sociological, or educational. Though regrettable, such acts of trespass are inevitable. Just as the law determines many of the conditions in which the doctor works, since he has responsibilities to the society in which he functions, so the psychiatrist cannot ignore the psychological origin and consequences of many legal beliefs, educational attitudes, and hospital and administrative routines.

1.2 Present Knowledge

It must be rare for decisions with serious coercive consequences to be taken with so little supporting evidence as in the case of juvenile delinquency. The inquirer who seeks by reading or discussion to ascertain current opinions on juvenile delinquency must be struck by the following two facts : first, each point of view, whether calmly or forcibly expressed, is based on a deep-rooted conviction ; and secondly, it is impossible to demonstrate objectively the validity of any one opinion.

There are many reasons for this lack of precise and objective knowledge. Because of the real difficulties of the subject, with its array of different factors to be taken into account, there are many chances of error creeping in, however scientific and conscientious the research worker may be. The subject does not lend itself to experimentation, and statistical procedures, such as the comparison between " normal " and " abnormal " groups, are full of pitfalls for the unwary. The emotional state in which workers and society approach the problem is even more responsible for this paucity of objective information, for the subject concerns our most fundamental and dearly-held sentiments, beliefs, morals, and traditions, and often unconsciously stirs up in us, both as individuals and as members of a group, long-buried feelings of guilt and aggression. Even the most scientific of workers, therefore, influenced either by his own emotional prejudices, or by those of his society, has difficulty in approaching the subject in an objective manner. The varied and often ambivalent opinions expressed either by individuals or by societies on the subject of punishment could well be used to prove this point.

These general remarks should not make us yield to an impotent scepticism ; on the contrary, they show the urgent need for the most objective research work possible. On the other hand, they also explain why, in this report, no final solution to the problem of juvenile delinquency has been offered. Rather, the aim has been to set out the problems, not to solve them, while at the same time underlining those isolated facts, which are already established, and such general theories, currently accepted, as seemed likely to further knowledge of the subject.

CHAPTER 2

ETIOLOGY OF JUVENILE DELINQUENCY

In the study of juvenile delinquency, psychiatry can contribute most substantially to the etiological aspect. In this report, therefore, particular attention will be given to this subject, though it is well to bear in mind that a survey of present knowledge is intended and not a detailed account of research work. At the risk of seeming tedious, I shall devote a section to general remarks on the growth of social adaptation in the normal child. Not that such a simplified account can be very instructive, but I felt the reader should be acquainted with the terminology employed so that the significance of the expressions used and the ideas defined in the subsequent sections could be better appreciated. Following this, I shall set out the main present-day psychiatric theories on the causes of juvenile delinquency. The section headings under which the various causal factors are brought together may appear arbitrary, but some abstraction and selection of material are necessary for a human study to be presented in readable form. Inevitably, any such selection is personal. Both reader and author must clearly understand the frame of reference used to interpret the facts of juvenile delinquency, which are so rich and varied that in interpreting them some distortion is inevitable. Both should realize, also, that other frames of reference could equally well be used.

Tappan's recent book [125] gives an excellent account of current theories on the causes of juvenile delinquency, and contains a comprehensive bibliography, comprising, however, almost exclusively, American works.

2.1 General Observations on Social Adaptation in the Normal Child

An impartial observer surveying the literature of the causes of juvenile delinquency will immediately note the contradictory nature of the opinions expressed by many learned and experienced workers. While some believe that a lack of social adaptation is due to constitutional, endogenous, and biological causes, others attribute it to accidental, external, and sociological causes.

Ahnsjö,[1] in his book on delinquent girls, gives a table which compares various writers' evaluation of the relative importance of endogenous and exogenous factors in the etiology of juvenile delinquency. The discrepancies revealed are striking. Some attribute 91%, others 12% to hereditary factors in the etiology of juvenile delinquency. Similarly, some writers assert that they have never seen a single case where external factors are alone responsible, compared with a figure of over 50% given by others.

Thus today, as in the nineteenth century, two age-old ideas clash: one of the " inborn criminal " linked with the name of Cesare Lombroso, the other, exemplified by the words of Victor Hugo : " the opening of a school is the closing of a prison ". Today these two opposing views have lost none of their pristine force, or striking power. They are, however, often disguised, may be more or less unconscious, and both can draw on more thorough and more scientific research work. Doubtless, many writers attempt a via media hoping to reconcile these opposing doctrines which may briefly be called the organic and the psychogenic approaches. Such an attempt is often merely on the surface and only serves to hide — even from its own advocate — a deep attachment to one or other point of view. Freud, however, with that biological approach so characteristic of his work, has already emphasized the importance of " somatic compliance ", although this idea has been sadly neglected by some of his followers. It is now forty years since Bleuler stressed that the correct question to ask when examining a behavioural phenomenon was not " is this organic or psychogenic ? " but " to what extent is this organic and to what extent is this psychogenic ? " Whenever behaviour and its origin are under discussion, his advice has the same value today as yesterday.

The two images, of " threshold " and " soil ", will help to clarify the problem.

The use of electric shock-therapy in psychiatry has proved anew that an epileptiform attack can occur in any individual, provided the current applied to the brain is strong enough, and has also shown that the strength of the current, sufficient to induce such an attack, varies from person to person. A patient suffering from idiopathic epilepsy (to use the medical term) can be thought of as having a brain which for one reason or another needs only a very weak electric current for a fit to occur : such a weak current would never result in a fit in a normal person. Another patient has a fit when his brain is stimulated by a cerebral tumour, or a fracture of the skull, though the brain of a third person would be inert to such stimuli. It appears, then, that each individual has a " threshold " of a certain height, which separates normal, localized, and controlled motor reactions from the uncontrolled and generalized response of the epileptic fit. A " normal " individual is one whose threshold is so high that only exceptionally strong stimuli can produce a fit, and an " epileptic " is one whose threshold is so low that even the normal stimuli of his metabolism may result in a fit. Between these two extremes, many intermediate stages exist, where thresholds of different heights are combined with stimuli of varying intensities. A similar process of reasoning can help to an understanding of certain hysterical states. During the war, men, who had never before shown signs of hysteria and have shown none since, developed hysterical symptoms after an intense psychic traumatic experience had suddenly overwhelmed their threshold level which under normal circumstances was sufficiently high to protect them from such reactions.

The idea of " soil " suggests an important point ; in the same way that arable land consists of the products of rock erosion together with the remains of vegetable matter which has grown there from seed brought from outside, so the biological " soil " of an individual contains not only hereditary and constitutional elements, but also the accumulating residue of life's numerous physical and psychological experiences. So it is that the concept of constitution transcends the narrow limits of hereditary characteristics and is both broader and more flexible. The ability of an individual constitution to come to terms with the ever-changing external world of today is in part due to these internalized and settled deposits of yesterday.

These two images, of " threshold " and stimulus, and of " soil " and seed, are particularly useful in explaining logically and accurately the genesis of social maladjustment. As Emerson confessed long ago, there was no crime or misdemeanour that had not tempted him at some time. Since then psycho-analysis — to mention only one method of introspection — has confirmed that in every individual there exist such antisocial leanings, against which defences are usually built to prevent their manifestation in primitive form. There are moments, however, when under continuous or temporary pressure these defences are overwhelmed, either permanently or momentarily, and lasting or transient delinquent behaviour ensues. In the child or the adolescent, even when perfectly normal, these defences are noticeably weaker than in the adult.

In the last fifty years, many workers have helped us understand why childhood and adolescence are periods particularly susceptible to social maladjustment. To obtain a thorough grasp of the peculiar nature of juvenile delinquency and of the psychological necessity for special legal and administrative procedures, it is important to master the findings of these workers on normal child development. I should like to give a brief account of present knowledge on this question, with special reference to the work of Anna Freud, and Piaget, though the work of Bühler, Gesell, Spitz, Stirnimann, Wolff, and many others should not be forgotten.

The child, at birth, is incomplete; large parts of his central nervous system are as yet undeveloped, and his mental activity is undifferentiated. He is a hedonist in that his activities, such as they are, aim at pleasure and the avoidance of pain. In feeding, evacuation, finger-sucking and other motor activities, as also in the progressive development of the reactions of attraction and repulsion, his whole behaviour at this period is the immediate and direct expression of instinctive urges. The baby blindly follows his biological needs, which give rise to a state of tension and a feeling of discomfort, and which he seeks to relieve. In the view of the modern psychologist, therefore, the child aims at comfort and pleasure so far as his limited physical powers permit him.

During the first months and years of life, the primitive and almost automatic mechanism of tension and relief from tension is changed by the increasing complexity of the ego. The progressive growth of sensory mechanisms, of memory, of an increasingly clear distinction between sensations originating within the body and those from the external world, of control over motor activity, of increasing awareness of his own, whole, personality, together with an ordering of his instinctive impulses, and not least, the acquisition of speech, all contribute to the formation and development of a small, organized, coherent, intelligible nucleus of personality. This nucleus, the centre of sensory perceptions, of conscious and rational behaviour, and the means of communication and of social adaptation, is known as the " ego ".

The ego so constituted, although still seeking to live by the " pleasure principle ", is progressively affected by the so-called " reality principle ". That is to say, the child, with ever increasing physical and intellectual skills, and greater emotional maturity, attempts gradually to adapt itself to the physical world and to fall in with the demands of adults and the conventions of society. The spontaneity, intensity, and extent of the instinctual satisfactions which the child allows itself are diminished; it is only at such a price that the child's feeling of inner security, so necessary to the growth of his personality, is assured.

There exists clearly, then, a link between the disturbances that can overtake the early development of the ego and the genesis of social maladjustment. It requires no imagination to envisage the social misdemeanours of a personality with the physical strength of an adult, but whose mental age is 8 or 9 months. The normal, progressive growth of the ego allows the child to feel secure in his instinctual behaviour, and also ensures his social security. In this sense, the normal development of the ego is of prime importance in a prophylactic approach to delinquency.

The demands of an organized society are but imperfectly met, however, at this early stage of development, since the child's ego is as yet weak and is at all times at the mercy of imperative instinctual urges. Furthermore, a code of behaviour based purely on an equilibrium of pleasure and reality principles will result in social difficulties, for a child will give way without further thought to a particular pattern of behaviour, once he has made certain that no unpleasant consequences will result. Adolescents who think they must not steal, only because they might be caught by the police, are examples of emotional development arrested at this stage.

To achieve a greater degree of social adaptation, thereby meeting yet further the demands of society, the child has to develop other capacities, a step forward which cannot occur without some degree of ego-development. He must now develop both the intellectual and emotional capacity for interpersonal relations. Such relations should evolve from the egocentric and parasitic stage, through a gradual socialization of thought and feeling, to a stage of mutual respect, of interchange of ideas and feelings, in short, of unselfish love, when to give is better than to receive. On the other hand, it must be made objectively possible for the child to experience in his immediate circle a deep, unfaltering, disinterested love, particularly from his mother or mother-substitute. This too is a slow, gradual evolution, illustrated in its earlier stages by the little girl's remark : " What's the use of loving Mummy and Daddy if they scold me just the same ? " The ultimate stages are attained only by the noblest characters. Between these two extremes all gradations of interpersonal relations can be found in the young child, both positive and negative, consecutively or simultaneously, and characterizing his relations with his mother, father, sisters, and brothers, his own small world, and society in general. This subtle interplay of " object relations " (as this emotional endowment of others has been called), of the resulting internal conflicts, and their resolution, gives rise to a new motive force in the personality—the super-ego. This super-ego is the product of the assimilation and incorporation by the child of all those moral precepts, in word or deed, given by his parents, or others who exercise in any way a parental role towards him.

Needless to say this new period in the child's development is of great importance to the growth of social adaptation. The child's capacity for emotional relations with others, and the code of morals which becomes second nature to him, complete the primal interplay of pleasure and reality principles and give to his behaviour all the qualities necessary for a normal life in society, particularly stability, security, and a steadfast spirit in temporary adversity.[a]

Piaget [90, 91, 92] has brought to light other factors which play a part in the child's social development. Briefly, he has called attention to the child's conception of reality, whereby till the age of 7 or 8 he tends to " reify ", that is to say he believes his conscious thoughts are independent objects outside himself. This is a universal characteristic of the child's mind to which moral ideas, with their scale of values, are no exception. For they are " reified " and endowed with an independent and almost physical existence, and are treated by the child as precepts imposed from without, independent of his moral judgement and beyond the reach of his own authority. In addition to this intellectual factor, Piaget describes an emotional factor—" adult coercion "—when an adult is seen as the repository of power and wisdom in proportion as he is the object of the child's love, fear, and transferred emotions. Hence, the adult's instructions, whether explicit or implicit, appear to the child as inescapable and compulsory.

The child's conception of reality and this factor of adult coercion, both interacting and working together, bring about a realistic moral sense. The child by his attitude towards reality treats as immutable and self-

---

[a] It is true, as the specialist knows, that the super-ego does not always further the development of social adaptation. In certain adverse situations the super-ego is of cardinal importance in the genesis of the psychoneuroses, and can hinder in a general way the maturation of the personality. There is not space to enlarge on these important points here, which are fully treated in recent psycho-analytic works.[64]

sufficient the adult's moral precepts and value judgements, which adult coercion obliges him to accept; thereby the child comes to believe that to be good is to obey adult commands, which carry the force of law, and to be naughty is to disobey. But how can a child most easily tell if his behaviour meets with the adult's approval? Parental reward or punishment will make it clear. The following rule results: right brings adult approval, wrong their punishment; with the corollary that what is not punished is not wrong. Piaget has shown by experiments how this habitual attitude of the child can lead to a code of morals, which to the adult appears paradoxical, and how such an attitude profoundly influences the child's good or bad behaviour as judged by adult standards.

Slowly the child's moral sense develops and assumes " normal " adult form by the progressive adaptation of his behaviour to society, and by the growth of mutual respect and co-operation, together with a code of personal ethics. Piaget has shown that only when the child feels from within the necessity to " do as you would be done by ", are feelings of mutual respect and a personal code developed. This theory, then, of the child's emotional growth is found to be similar to the one previously described, but originates from a slightly different school of thought. Given the normal development of all these factors, the child has at its disposal the psychological means for a good social adaptation, and, although this adaptation may be menaced by puberty and adolescence, once these periods are safely past it will bring about, sooner or later, that inner stability which allows a further harmonious integration into society.

This brief survey might lead to misunderstandings were it to be read by an uninitiated public, who need more than a mere summary of the main facts. Two points, however, need to be emphasized: (1) the development just described is not without its ups and downs; the various stages overlap, progress may be delayed or halted, partly or completely, temporarily or permanently, which makes the theoretical curve of moral growth uncertain and irregular; (2) as with nations, whose history explains certain traits in their present behaviour, so in the individual later behaviour contains traces of earlier growth processes. Under certain conditions a permanent or temporary regression to behaviour long outgrown can suddenly or gradually occur. The younger the child and the more recent his acquisition of good social behaviour, the more frequent and disastrous are his regressions to earlier levels of behaviour which occur with an ease rare in the normal adult.

In this section I have discussed those biological and psychological factors which render the child and adolescent particularly liable to antisocial behaviour, and I have tried to explain why it is easier for the young than for the adult to cross unawares the narrow boundary which separates social maladjustment from delinquency.

2.2 Sociological Factors

All those factors which are primarily related to the external environment, and which do not involve any complicated psychological mechanisms, will be classified here as sociological. It will, however, be necessary at the end of this section to review this over-simplified statement which here serves merely as a starting-point for discussion.

Certain easily verifiable facts at first sight seem to indicate that a large percentage of juvenile delinquents do not show any obvious signs of mental or physical illness.

For example, in 1947, of the 7,000 juveniles appearing before the Chicago juvenile courts, 705 or only 10% were referred to psychiatric examination. Similarly in Lausanne (Switzerland) where there is a close collaboration between the juvenile court and child psychiatrists, the average proportion of cases referred for medical and psychological examination for the years 1947-1949 was 12%. It is likely that the statistics of other cities, possessing the necessary facilities for the psychiatric examination of juvenile delinquents, would yield similar results. It is, of course, highly probable that the magistrates do not recognize all the cases which need psychiatric examination, and it is very desirable that a higher proportion should be thus examined, both in the interests of justice and to obtain improved methods of psychological re-education. Nevertheless, a comparison between the total number of juvenile delinquents and the number who show marked signs of psychiatric, or any other, illness seems to prove that the majority of juveniles appearing for whatever reason before the juvenile courts, or their equivalents, are medically normal. Statistical tables of the incidence of crime supply further evidence, and a comparison between the number of delinquents in years of political and social peace with the number in years of unrest shows that the incidence of juvenile crime varies with social factors. Thus, in Finland the numbers of juveniles aged 15-18 appearing before the courts were: 1945, 6,545; 1946, 5,129; 1947, 4,451; 1948, 4,072. While the statistics for the incidence of crime during the war and the post-war years need to be interpreted with caution because of numerous changes in law, the variable efficiency of the police, and an elastic interpretation of what constituted an offence, it is generally agreed in most European countries and in America that the war had a definite effect on the spread of juvenile delinquency, but that its influence is now decreasing in most countries. Similar observations had already been made in the first World War (for further details see Exner,[30] Grassberger,[50] and Bolterauer[8]). It seems difficult to maintain that these thousands of extra juvenile delinquents, who for a few years, in every country, thronged the courts, were all suffering from serious psychological disorders, breaking out in the first years of the war, only to disappear once the war ended. Such a theory is even less admissible if one considers that the psychological factors active in delinquency, and especially the constitutional factors, have often a long incubation, and delayed effects. A more plausible theory is that this sudden and temporary increase in juvenile delinquency is due to external circumstances, which affect the personality as an accident might, rather than deeply, like an illness. In the work already mentioned by Grassberger[50] on the rates and kinds of recidivism, this point is convincingly and brilliantly established.

In fact, in addition to the examples just given, the part played by social factors in the etiology of juvenile delinquency has been repeatedly demonstrated, with the result that some sociologists have gone so far as to assert that juvenile delinquency is essentially due to the action of a variable number of external events on a normal personality.

Among the more recent and authoritative books on the sociological aspects of this problem Sellin's [111] is to be noted. This book contains first, a detailed and critical examination of the sources of error in previous sociological research work, and secondly a plan for sociological research. Shaw [112, 113, 114, 115] of Chicago, the author of a number of books on this problem, is now director of the "Chicago Area Project", which has as its hypothesis that a high proportion of delinquency in children is due to the social conditions in which they are brought up, and which seeks to remedy this situation by securing the co-operation of the affected families through their own desire to improve their living conditions.

Young [139, 140] has published two particularly interesting studies on the families of the Russian Molokans sect which emigrated to Los Angeles between 1905 and 1908. She found that in these families within 22 years the incidence of juvenile delinquency rose from 5% to 80% of the total juvenile population, although the ethnic constitution of the stock remained unchanged.

Similarly, the concentration of juvenile delinquency in urban areas and its comparative rarity in country areas should be remembered. [29, 117] Further evidence of the importance of social factors can be found in the work of Burt,[19] now a classic, and also in the publications of Carr-Saunders, Mannheim & Rhodes [20] and of Mannheim.[81]

It is not possible here either to give a detailed analysis of these works, or to determine the exact percentage of delinquents in whom the main etiological factors are social. It is, however, necessary to stress the weight of evidence which proves that a large percentage of the children and adolescents appearing before the courts are neither physically nor psychologically seriously ill. Applying the principle of "threshold" as outlined in the introduction, it would seem as if these delinquents have a threshold perhaps a little lower than their contemporaries, but which under normal circumstances would have been high enough. They have, however, had to face such adverse circumstances that only a much higher threshold could have prevented a delinquent outbreak. Furthermore, the ratio between these almost normal juveniles and those with major psychological disorders varies with time and place. As a general rule, when times are quiet, community life peaceful, and the standard of living high, the delinquent population contains proportionately few such "normals". On the other hand, when community life is unsettled (as in times of strife, war, postwar, revolutions, mass unemployment, major industrial changes), when the mean standard of living is low (as in some big European towns), when social unrest is allied with poor economic conditions (as in some big American cities where immigration constantly changes the population, giving a special character to the poverty peculiar to large cities), then the number of "normals" who are the victims of these disturbed times increases considerably. This must be one of the reasons why different authorities do not emphasize to the same extent the part played by social factors in the etiology of juvenile delinquency. Some observers, owing to the time and place in which they work, have never had the opportunity of witnessing the mobilization and the deployment of this mass of latent delinquents, so aptly called " the reserve troops of juvenile delinquency ".

As already stated, the psychiatrist is asked to see on the average only 10% of juvenile court cases. This is much too low a figure and implies that the psychiatrist sees only the more psychopathic delinquents. As a result he is led to generalize about all delinquents from this small sample, which being specially selected distorts his picture of the whole. Some magistrates and re-educators fall into the opposite error. Faced, day in day out, with a constant stream of delinquents, normal and abnormal, they tend to underestimate both the quantitative and the qualitative aspects of these psychologically disturbed cases. These cases are only too apt to dismay those seeking to assess or re-educate them, using only their common sense. Magistrates or re-educators find methods which are usually successful to be useless here, and hence do not like to dwell on this type of case, minimizing its importance in comparison with the large numbers of juveniles who respond favourably to simple and classical measures. Since, therefore, the psychiatrist on the one hand, and the magistrates on the other, are often not talking about the same type of case, there is a clash of opinions, which is serious, since frequently it interferes with close, co-operative work.

Although recent personal experience, reinforced by this investigation, obliges me as a psychiatrist to take special note of this group of delinquents conveniently classified as " non-psychiatric delinquents ", certain reservations must be made. Although psychological factors need not be the primary determinants of a delinquent act, such an act, like any other piece of human behaviour, cannot, nevertheless, take place without involving the psyche. If a social factor is to become a criminal force, it must set in motion a number of psychological processes. The ease with which such processes are set in motion depends on the previous organization of the subject's personality, his constitution, his life experience, his resistances, and his weaknesses. The psychiatrist B. Glueck once strikingly remarked (personal communication from S. Glueck) " a factor cannot be a cause before it is a motive ". Neither the psychiatrist nor the psychologist, therefore, can neglect these sociological cases, and despite all that has been said, both by others and by myself, it would be of great value if juveniles belonging to this group were to be examined both medically and psychologically.

Finally, even the " normal " delinquent (the word " normal " being now used with newly learnt caution), and perhaps even more than the " abnormal " delinquent, in appearing before a court and in being subsequently labelled " delinquent " may suffer a psychological trauma, the effects of which are reinforced by later measures taken about him. From then on he becomes less " normal " and grows more like those other cases needing psychiatric help.

2.3 Somatic and Constitutional Factors

Since this report serves a practical purpose, somatic and constitutional factors have been deliberately brought together in this section to survey simultaneously their causal relation to juvenile delinquency. It is, however, realized that these two terms are both very vague and difficult to define and also that the somatic is not necessarily constitutional and vice versa. Nevertheless, these two terms are often linked together in the minds of workers in delinquency, probably because they imply the existence of factors which are considered, rightly or wrongly, to be beyond modification, and to bind their subjects to an unalterable and fatal state of moral weakness. To avoid confusion, this close connexion between the soma and the constitutional will be maintained here.

2.3.1 *Constitutional psychopaths*

There are few psychiatric ideas more in dispute today than that of constitutional psychopathy and its relation to difficulties in social adaptation. At the recent 27th Congress of the American Association of Orthopsychiatry,[b] despite a lively discussion led by D. M. Levy, H. S. Lippman, R. Lourie, L. G. Lowrey, L. A. Lurie, and R. Rabinovitch, the various opposing points of view remained unreconciled.

Lombroso first put forward and championed the idea of a constitutional delinquency in his famous book *L'Uomo delinquente* (1876), an idea which he later modified and developed. His theories were adopted not only by other Italian criminologists including di Tullio,[128] to mention one contemporary exponent amongst others, but also by many criminologists in other countries, notably Vervaeck,[132] in Belgium, Hooton [61] in America, and others.

To examine these works in any detail would be quite outside the scope and aims of this report. Comment must be limited to the statement that Lombroso's idea of a specific psychosomatic type of born criminal is today generally held to be without foundation. This should not, however, lead us to forget the great debt owed to Lombroso and his followers for attempting to give to criminal studies a biological basis. Father Gemelli [39] — though no follower of Lombroso — has aptly written: the great merit of Lombroso is that " he stressed the need in delinquent studies to leave the narrow and necessarily abstract paths of the law for the study of individuals and their behaviour". Lombroso, thereby, became the father of modern criminology, and even when the latter rejects his doctrines it does so in the name of the revolutionary principles he put forward three-quarters of a century ago. Similarly, Vervaeck, to mention only one contemporary follower, has been most influential in Belgium in securing reforms in the penal code and in prisons, which have made his country one of the most advanced today.

What today is meant exactly by the term " constitutional psychopath "? There seems to be no general agreement on the accepted meaning of the term. As used by some European schools [69] of thought, as well as in

---

[b] This congress met in Atlantic City, N.J., from 22 to 24 February 1950.

America, it appears to be restricted to patients whose behaviour is definitely antisocial and who have other well-defined characteristics. It is agreed that they are "egocentric", "unable to profit by experience", "emotionally unstable", "lacking in feeling", etc. White [134] writes "the latter label [psychopathic personality] is generally applied when the following characteristics are present: habitual delinquent behaviour, a marked lack of moral scruples, insensitivity to the rights of others, and a generally erratic and purposeless way of living". Similar ideas are expressed by Lauretta Bender's [5] use of the word, in her well-known paper in which she attacks the hypothesis of the constitutional origin of a psychopath.

With reference to these views, the German and Swiss schools of psychiatry originally responsible for introducing this term into the psychiatrist's vocabulary (following Koch's work in 1891) give to the word "psychopathic" a wider, yet more precise, meaning. Schneider,[110] in 1923, made an important contribution to the definition of its nosology with the now classic phrase: "a psychopathic personality is an abnormal personality suffering under his abnormality or causing suffering to society". Luxenburger [78] has also neatly written: "the symptomatology of a psychopath consists of a variable number of behavioural patterns which are sufficiently unusual or unnecessary to disturb the harmonious relations between the individual and his environment, and lead to suffering within the individual, and to the individual inflicting suffering on those around him".

Although these are but descriptive definitions, they imply an etiological hypothesis, that psychopathic behaviour—in contradistinction to psychoneurotic behaviour or to behaviour secondary to an acquired organic illness—has a constitutional basis and belongs therefore to the group of traits which are a fundamental and integral part of the personality.

This, then, is my final definition: psychopathic traits are permanent character abnormalities, of constitutional origin, which are not derived either from psychoses, neuroses, or mental deficiency, and which predispose the psychopathic personality to behavioural disorders from which he suffers or causes society to suffer.

The point to be stressed is that this concept of psychopathic personality in no way defines or delimits the kind of behaviour which is "unusual and unnecessary". Schneider himself advocated a non-systematized classification of psychopathy based solely on the main symptom in each case. Although he describes ten different psychopathic types, he does not seem to treat his classification otherwise than as a first approximation, essentially practical and didactic in nature. Clearly then, the restricted use of the term "constitutional psychopaths" to include only those who are "delinquent, without moral scruples, insensitive", etc., as is the common practice in the USA, gives to these words a quite different meaning from the one they possess in the country of their origin where much work has been done on their underlying concepts. To the continental European psychiatrist the term "psychopath" in no way implies a delinquent. Indeed some psychopaths (for example depressives, abulics, neurasthenics) are by their very nature rarely likely to commit delinquent acts. Furthermore, to believe that delinquency, as such, including its component aspects of the law, society, and the police, can become an hereditary biological characteristic is an absurdity which no previous upholder of the idea of constitutional psychopathic personality has ever thought of advancing.

It was necessary to specify and to clarify these issues, so that, a clear-cut attitude having been adopted, the problem of the relations between constitutional psychopathy and juvenile delinquency could be raised as follows: does one find individuals with permanent and apparently unalterable character disorders which are significantly linked to hereditary and constitutional factors? Can such disorders influence social adaptation? What are the current answers to these questions?

To simplify the problem, consider first the theoretical aspects. There is no valid reason for refusing to admit at least the possibility that constitutional and hereditary factors can so influence character formation as to predispose some individuals to delinquent behaviour. Since it is agreed that hereditary and constitutional factors can determine to some extent height, body-build, and, in psychology, intelligence level, why then may they not have an important influence upon character? What is perhaps more surprising is the number of writers today who appear in fact to deny even this theoretical possibility. Their attitude would seem to be due to prejudices, both emotional and ideological, which are also often unconscious.

This theoretical possibility does not prove that such cases actually do occur, or that they occur in numbers sufficiently great to warrant all the nosological importance given to them by various writers. It is precisely on this latter point that opinions differ.

For instance, Sutherland [124] has pointed out that in the States of Massachusetts and New York, psychiatric reports show that 10% of the prisoners are psychopaths, while for the same period in the State of Illinois 75% were so diagnosed: such a discrepancy is more likely to be due to the psychiatrist than to the prisoners. Some doctors have made too free use of the diagnosis "constitutional psychopath" and have thus helped to bring the term into discredit. The psychiatrist, finding that his patients' abnormal personality traits do not respond to his therapeutic efforts, concludes that this must be because they are constitutional, and, since they are constitutional, naturally the patient cannot be cured. It is thus easy to see to what depths of therapeutic nihilism such a " petitio principii " leads. It is also equally unwarranted to try to deny the existence of constitutional character disorders only on the grounds that some practitioners have found therein a pretext for laziness.

Consider next the data of neurophysiology and of modern studies in genetics. Recent advances in knowledge of the normal and pathological functioning of the vegetative nervous system seem clearly to show that constitutional factors are concerned in the formation of character, and hence indirectly of delinquency. The work of Eppinger & Hess, and the brilliant studies of the Swiss physiologist, W. R. Hess [56, 57, 58] have opened the way to new advances and to many new hypotheses concerning psychosomatic correlations, the richness and variety of which will become increasingly important.

Although electro-encephalographic studies exploring the higher mental functions and their disorders are still tentative, some workers have already been able to obtain some extremely interesting information on the somatic components of mental behaviour. (See, for example, the recent work by Hill & Parr.[60])

Mention must also be made of work in recent years on prenatal and birth conditions likely to affect the central nervous system, particularly the studies of the Rhesus factor, of toxic foetal states, and of the anatomical and physiological traumata at birth [c] with their sequelae.[116]

There are many genetic studies on the inheritance of antisocial character traits, particularly in Germany, among these the most numerous being comparative studies of criminal tendencies in identical and non-identical twins. Lange,[73] the best known of these workers, found 10 delinquent pairs in 13 pairs of identical twins, compared with 2 pairs in 17 pairs of non-identical twins.

Later investigations, notably by Stumpfl,[123] Kranz,[70] Rosanoff, Handy & Rosanoff,[106] have all shown, though to a lesser extent than was found by Lange, a higher incidence of delinquency in identical than in non-identical twins. Guttmacher[54] together with many other Americans, including Healy & Bronner,[55] using a number of psychological and biological arguments, deny the validity of these researches, pointing out that they contain many sources of error. On the other hand, a great number of geneticists, despite these sources of error (and Kranz in discussing his results has taken them into account), hold that these investigations prove their point, and show that constitutional factors are of importance in social maladaptation, a conclusion which finds support in the published proceedings of the International Congress of Psychiatry, held in Paris, in 1950.[62]

---

[c] Dr. Somersalo, at the children's clinic of Professor Ylppö, in Helsinki, is finishing an important study of the late sequelae following the use of forceps.

It seems to me that this disagreement arises from the critics of genetic studies accusing the geneticist of believing that delinquent behaviour is itself inherited. It is, therefore, necessary to point out once again that no serious geneticists have ever held this view, and that they believe only they have shown, as a real and important fact, the inheritance of a number of character tendencies which together predispose to delinquent behaviour.

Turning now to the clinical evidence: in the first place, the work of Kretschmer in Germany, and Sigaud in France, with their forerunners and their pupils, must be mentioned. These workers, and many others working along the same lines, have accumulated a great deal of evidence which clearly shows a positive correlation between body-build and certain personality traits, a result which simultaneously implies a correlation between these traits and inherited and constitutional factors.

Recently, Sheldon [116] has sought to create a new anthropometric technique for delinquency, but his results to date, although well documented and illustrated by a wealth of photographs, have not gained the support of the majority of American specialists.

If current psychiatric and medical experience are considered next, it seems impossible that a psychiatrist, however keen an advocate of psychotherapy, could deny that he has met a large number of cases of behavioural disorders which have impressed him by their constant pattern of behaviour and their resistance to all forms of treatment. When also, as is possible in small countries, entire families are followed up for years and the behavioural disorder of each member is found to have a similar and unchanging pattern, the hypothesis of the constitutional origin of such disorders is particularly apt.

It is quite true that there are patients diagnosed as psychopaths who recover either spontaneously or through some new, clever, and persistent method of treatment, thereby showing the reversible nature of their condition, which cannot therefore be constitutional. Lindner [76] in his book gives a good illustration of this point. But such cases are exceptional and can serve only to make psychiatrists even more cautious in using the diagnosis of psychopath.

Amongst criminologists, Frey [33, 34, 35] of Basle (Switzerland), over a number of years, has published a series of articles, soon to appear in book form, in which, as a result of his experiences with juvenile courts and of his careful and detailed investigations, he also comes to the conclusion that there is a group, though small, of constitutional psychopathic delinquents with well marked features.

A few additional remarks are necessary to give precision to this all too brief summary.

(1) People do not inherit ready-made behaviour patterns, but more or less marked general tendencies, some being stronger than others. Hence it is completely wrong to speak of " inherited delinquency ". What can be inherited is temperament and certain

tendencies of character, which, in particular circumstances, whether individual or social, favour the later appearance of delinquent behaviour. If the reader refers to the idea of "soil", and its slow formation, as defined earlier (page 13), he will immediately understand how heredity and environment can result in the long run in the formation of a delinquent character type.

(2) Especially in the field of psychological predispositions there are good reasons for believing that the inheritance of tendencies is a recessive one. Thus, for a tendency to appear it must be inherited from both sides of the family, the children of the same parents not necessarily having the same tendencies; it may jump one, or several, generations; it may completely disappear; or it may make its appearance—within a minimum of two generations—through the introduction of outside genes. It is, therefore, abundantly clear that the possible combinations are great and that the laws governing these combinations can be discovered only by genetic studies conducted on a vast scale with the greatest scientific care.

(3) Criminologists using the term "constitutional psychopath" should bear in mind that psychiatrists often make this diagnosis because the patient has shown consistently antisocial behaviour since early childhood. If the non-medical criminologist, when investigating the behaviour of juveniles thus diagnosed, discovers that they are very resistant to all re-educational measures, and that the strength of their resistances seems to be proportional to the duration of their antisocial behaviour, he must beware of the fallacy in logic of "petitio principii", or begging the question. In fact, these delinquents are not psychopaths because they are so difficult to re-educate, but they have been so diagnosed by doctors because their re-education has proved till now impossible.

(4) Although the following argument has little scientific merit, the idea of constitutional psychopathy has frequently been criticized on the grounds of being negative and leading to therapeutic nihilism. While it is true that the idea of the word constitutional psychopathy leaves little room for cures in the strict medical sense, it facilitates the adoption of a number of social measures which can considerably alleviate the psychopath's lot and even lead to improved social adjustment. In this connexion Schneider's definition (see page 22) is particularly helpful. All psychiatrists interested in social problems and all psychiatric social workers know of the beneficial results obtained in the most therapeutically difficult psychopaths by a change of environment. If, then, the use of the diagnosis "psychopath" results in beneficial social procedures, rather than in numerous years of costly and laborious psychotherapy or in fruitless attempts at re-education which only discourage re-educator and pupil, it no longer seems reasonable to stress the negative aspects of this term.

In view of the negative attitude of many psychiatrists towards the concept of "constitutional psychopath" it was important to spend some time unravelling the various misunderstandings that exist about it, in order to show not only that it is a theoretical possibility, but also that there is much evidence for the existence of an important number of delinquency cases belonging to this category, and to show finally that this concept offers good opportunities for applying rational measures to soften the fate of these cases while protecting the interests of society.

2.3.2 *Mental deficiency*

Pearce,[89] when discussing the more-generally accepted factors in juvenile delinquency, wrote: "A great deal is known about the influence of intelligence in juvenile delinquency. It seems definite that the intelligence of the average delinquent is considerably less than that of his non-delinquent neighbour." Goddard,[45] who appears the most dogmatic on this point, goes so far as to say that the presence of mental defect will of itself explain a delinquent's behaviour. Burt [19] states " ... my own percentage... reveals among the delinquent population a proportion of mental defectives five times as great as among the school population at large. Mental defect, beyond all controversy, therefore, is a notable factor in the production of crime. " Glueck & Glueck [41, 43] in their work have come to the same conclusion.

In opposition to this view, which is shared by many other authors, there are a number of recent publications where the contrary view is put forward. For instance, Stein, psychiatrist to the Chicago Juvenile Court, in a yet unpublished study of 705 juvenile delinquents seen by him in 1947, states that his findings show that in all probability the distribution of intelligence amongst juveniles labelled delinquents is the same as, if not higher than, for non-delinquents. Ramer, [98] investigating in Stockholm the records of the pupils in classes for mentally retarded children, arrives at the same conclusions.

Sutherland, [124] in a critical evaluation of the results of 175,000 intelligence tests given to American delinquents from 1910 to 1928, believes that the methods used are so unstandardized and contain so many technical errors as to cast doubt on the value of the test results.

For example, the test results for 1910-1914 show that 50% of American prisoners were mentally defective, compared with 20% for 1925-1928. As Sutherland correctly remarks, it is more likely that the methods of test administration have changed between 1910-1925 than that the intelligence level should have risen so strikingly.

He therefore concludes that this analysis shows the correlation between delinquency and mental deficiency to be, on the whole, relatively weak.

Clara Chassell [21] concludes her detailed survey of the literature "the relation is positive but low ".

The conclusion of the classic work by Healy & Bronner [55] contains the remark " intellectual level [does] not, in general, distinguish the delinquent from his non-delinquent sibling, though [it] may have importance... in the individual case ".

Exner [30] also holds that the correlation between mental deficiency and delinquency is barely significant, and by no means implies a relation of cause and effect.

Here, then, is one of the problems on which opinions vary widely, as was mentioned in the introduction. To get a clearer view of the situation further research is required, taking into account all possible sources of error, especially the methods of selecting delinquents for testing, the selection of control groups, the methods of test administration, and the influence of the emotions on the intelligence level. It would also be valuable to know if the new, and more appropriate, teaching methods, now in use with backward children, are successful in helping their later social adjustment, a hypothesis which can be inferred from Ramer's work.[96]

It would also be reasonable to expect that whenever the " reserve troops of delinquency " are either partially or totally mobilized, for whatever reason, a number of mental defectives will be found in the ranks owing to their mental instability and suggestibility. (See page 19.)

Three further points should be made: the first practical, the second methodological, the third theoretical:

(1) Whatever the order of correlation between mental defect and delinquency, it is now generally agreed that a mentally defective delinquent has a poorer prognosis than a delinquent of average intelligence.[d] Furthermore, the treatment of these mental defectives is a special, and often difficult, problem. It would be necessary to segregate them in specially designed schools, where appropriate treatment could be carried out, thereby considerably lightening the burden of the personnel in reform institutions for delinquents of normal intelligence.

(2) The often artificial nature of the delinquent group selected must be borne in mind when undertaking studies of the correlation between social maladjustment and intelligence levels. For instance, the inmates of a reform institution for juvenile delinquents are clearly an unsuitable group to select, since magistrates avoid sending intelligent delinquents for residential treatment and prefer to try either probation or boarding-out. Also the unintelligent delinquents have a greater tendency to recidivism (Exner [30]) and hence are proportionately more numerous in reform institutions. Finally, many intelligent juvenile delinquents never come before the courts, either because their parents have successfully cut short any inquiry, or because, by reason of their intelligence, the crimes are committed in such a way that their perpetrators are never discovered.[136]

(3) If the reader refers, at the beginning of this section, to the broad survey of the child's personality development, and of the various phases in his social adaptation, it will be seen that ego-formation leading to super-ego development, and on to successful social adaptation, depends largely on intellectual factors, a point clearly shown by Anna Freud [32] in her work on ego-development, and recently brilliantly proved anew by Germaine Guex.[53] Theoretically then, a correlation between intelligence and satisfactory social adaptation can reasonably be predicted, were it not that the situation is complicated by many other factors, which tend to cancel out the effects of mental deficiency. Thus, those emotional needs of the child

---

[d] See especially Glueck & Glueck.[45] Healy & Bronner [46] do not agree with this opinion.

which help him to identify his conduct with the moral code of his parents are frequently particularly strong in mentally defective children who, because of their mental defect, greatly need the support of their environment. On the other hand, a certain level of intelligence is required to commit a crime, hence not only idiots and imbeciles, but also some mental defectives, are excluded from delinquency.

2.3.3 *Organic disease and illness*

It is somewhat ironic to find some magistrates and re-educators, though most unwilling to take psychiatry into account, immediately giving way before an organic disease or illness, as if faced by some magical power, and granting these patients an almost absolute immunity from punishment. For instance, Article 13 of the Swiss penal code states :

" If the accused is deaf and dumb, or if it is alleged that he is epileptic, he will be so examined " (i.e., his mental state will be examined).

Further on, the same code obliges the authorities to give special treatment to a child or adolescent who is " blind, deaf and dumb, or epileptic " (Articles 86 and 92).

But all who are familiar with juvenile delinquency know that such cases are rare today and of little importance in the overall picture in the psychopathology of crime. M. Jeanneret, Chairman of the Geneva juvenile court, has told me that there have been no deaf and dumb or epileptic cases before his court in the last eight years, when the new penal code was introduced. Of the 7,000 juvenile delinquents brought before the Chicago juvenile court in 1947, Stein, psychiatrist to the court, found only 12 cases of epilepsy and 13 who were " hard of hearing ".

These remarks do not, however, apply to the contribution of " epileptiform " personalities to social maladjustment, a subject to be discussed later.

There exist various papers of doubtful scientific value, claiming to establish a correlation between tuberculosis, malaria, or other similar endemic diseases, and delinquency ; I mention this here only for the sake of completeness. These correlations are derived from the figures of the incidence of these illnesses in juvenile delinquents and their parents, while no attempt is made to discover, with equal thoroughness and with the same techniques, their incidence in a control group of non-delinquents, with similar sociological backgrounds. It is greatly to be regretted that workers continue to devote time, which must appear valuable to them, on such superficial work.

For a long time much emphasis was placed on syphilis, especially congenital syphilis, particularly by the French school, as a causative and psychopathological factor in delinquency. This point of view has been recently advocated by Brantmay [18] amongst others. Most authorities today, however, in France and elsewhere, do not attach much importance to the part played by this social disease in the causation of juvenile delinquency, without of course denying that in an individual case it may be important. Juvenile general paralysis, the only clear-cut congenital syphilitic condition found in children, for all practical purposes does not give rise to any medico-legal problems, since these patients are generally so markedly mentally defective that they are incapable of committing an offence.

There are certain chronic illnesses and physical disabilities which produce various psychological reactions in their victims, as, for instance, over-compensation for inferiority feelings (described by the Adlerian school,[e] among others) and these in turn may lead to reactive antisocial behaviour. But this is rather more a question of psychogenesis, than of primary somatogenesis.

Research work on the physiopathology of the central nervous system, and especially of the autonomic nervous system, enriched by recent information on the immediate and the far-reaching effects of leucotomy, and other psychosurgical operations, forces consideration of the possible influence of organic disease of the central nervous system on a predisposition to delinquency, particularly where disorders of emotional control and of loss of mental inhibition are concerned.

If the illness or disability occurs before birth, at birth, or in very early infancy, it belongs more to the category of constitutional psychopathies described above. If, however, it occurs at a later date, it must be considered as a possible causative factor, and this is especially true of the various forms of encephalitis which today are known to occur more frequently than had previously been supposed, as complications of the infectious diseases of childhood, though often unrecognized.

The severe personality disturbances following head injuries in adults are well known, and similar traumatic consequences are often quoted as an explanation, particularly in non-medical circles, for behavioural disorders in children. Mention must, therefore, be made of a number of papers (by Riggenbach,[105] Lutz,[77] Probst,[96] and others) which show that the effects of head injuries in children, even though serious at the time of the injury, are in the majority of cases remarkably benign and transitory.

Mention must now be made of one special group of disorders, the " epileptoid " (or " ixophrenia " of Strömgen). There is reason to hope that one day the electro-encephalogram will enable this group to be defined more precisely as a nosological entity. Although the etiology of this disorder remains obscure, certain " epileptoid " features commonly recur, particularly impulsiveness, and a kind of viscosity in their emotional and intellectual reactions which predispose them to delinquent behaviour. They do not have motor attacks, or their equivalents, but the electro-encephalograph contains wave and spike tracings typical of epilepsy.

---

[e] An excellent general account of Adlerian doctrines will be found in the book by Madelaine Ganz.[38] See also Wexberg.[133]

ETIOLOGY

It is by now clear from this brief account that the organic diseases and illnesses important in the genesis of delinquency cannot be limited to blindness, deaf-mutism, or overt epilepsy. Another conclusion is that the importance and exact part to be attributed to these organic factors is as yet uncertain. It would seem, in general, that they are not among the most important causative factors in delinquency. It is possible that further research into the physiopathology of the nervous system will modify this opinion. In any case today, it can be said that, although it is a wise principle to have all epileptic, blind, and deaf-mute delinquents, as well as those suspected of tuberculosis or syphilis, medically examined, such examinations can add little of practical importance to the knowledge, treatment, and prevention of juvenile delinquency. To limit the psychiatrist's work to the examination and treatment of these cases is not a particularly happy way of recognizing his speciality.

2.4 Disturbances in the Psychological Development of the Personality

In this section, I shall bring together the various psychological factors which, by their influence on the personality of the child or adolescent, can disturb his social adjustment, and hence perhaps make a delinquent of him. The possible effects of these factors has been studied now for a long time, and since the first papers of Freud, almost contemporaneous with those of Janet in France, the psychological interpretation of social maladjustment has grown considerably in importance. Certain chapters in the works of Adler, perhaps too often neglected today, constitute a contribution of permanent value to the understanding of juvenile antisocial behaviour.[38, 133] Aichhorn[2] was the first to apply, in a scientific and practical way, the knowledge gained from depth psychology to the diagnosis and treatment of juvenile delinquency. No praise can be too great for the work of this brilliant teacher and masterly psycho-analyst, who opened the way to all the modern conceptions in the study and treatment of juvenile delinquents. Since then there have been numerous publications, among which Käthe Friedländer's[37] deserves special mention for its didactic value. The following section, then, is based on the teachings of Aichhorn, as he expounded them in a course of lectures to the Office médico-pédagogique vaudois at Lausanne, Switzerland, in 1948. Even more than before in this report, the need to be concise must result in over-simplification.

2.4.1 *Qualitative defects in the super-ego*

If the reader will bear in mind the outline of the formation of the personality given at the beginning of this section, it will be easy to understand what can happen if the moral precepts, which the child seeks to incorporate at the time of the formation of the superego, are antisocial, or even criminal. The child's super-ego, although developed in the normal way, will contain elements which will lead to antisocial behaviour. In other words, the delinquent's personality has a normal structure, is built according to the everyday laws of psychology, but the material used for his super-ego was borrowed from antisocial personalities, and hence renders him liable to antisocial behaviour and in certain circumstances to delinquency.

> One could almost, therefore, speak here of a normal personality, and strictly speaking it would have been possible to include these cases in the group of delinquents from social causes. This has not been done because, in this type of case, the primary antisocial environmental force results in the formation of a relatively stable psychological structure, the super-ego, whose content cannot be changed for the better either easily or quickly. Hence this social cause of delinquency expresses itself as a profound psychological deformation of the personality, and for this reason it seemed best to include these cases here.

In more practical terms, this type of case is found among the children of antisocial parents, or in antisocial communities such as exist in certain neighbourhoods in big cities. But it must be remembered that a great many other children brought up in such surroundings have normal, or almost normal, super-egos. There is no room here to discuss this finding, which must have both biological and psychological causes.

2.4.2 *Partial retardation in development*

If the reader refers once more to my outline of personality development, it will be apparent that it is the result of a series of separate stages of growth, of gradual acquisition, as much sensory as motor, intellectual and emotional. Each separate stage fits into the whole, like stones in a wall. If growth, in one or more directions, does not coincide with the growth of the whole, instability results and normal development in other directions may even be delayed: much as the absence of one or two stones will diminish the strength of a whole building and even prevent its normal structural completion. Numerous examples of such retardation in development can be found in any of the varied aspects of child care. Paediatricians and teachers are well versed in the consequences of these retardations. The following examples must suffice here.

Irregularities in the child's emotional growth in the first months and early years of life may compromise the building of the ego more or less seriously. Since to go into the full details here would take too long, it is enough to stress the serious consequences that often follow any disturbance in the normal child-mother relationship. Many paediatricians (for example Stirnimann [122]) have long been aware that the infant is no mere digestive tube, as paediatricians used to assert in the heyday of feeding schedules, but is a being with a mental life, both intellectual and emotional, capable of increasingly differentiated reactions to both favourable and unfavourable atmospheres. A great deal of recent work has produced precise data on the importance of the psychological conditions of the early years of growth. Two authors in particular should be mentioned: Goldfarb [46, 47, 48] with his study of the intellectual development of children brought up in institutions, and Spitz,[120, 121] who through his detailed, psycho-analytic study of infants brought up at home or in institutions, has become the chief exponent of the view that the quality of the early relationship between mother and child is a determining factor in the later development of the personality. Bowlby [16] in a recent paper, and from an entirely different starting-point, has also arrived at the conclusion that emotional disturbance in early infancy is one of the most specific factors, though naturally not the only one, in the causation of juvenile delinquency. Bowlby,[17] on the initiative of WHO, is at present preparing an extremely important and detailed report to substantiate this hypothesis, which is empirically shared by most psychiatrists, and, I should like to stress, by most re-educators with whom I discussed the matter. Lauretta Bender [5] whose work has already been mentioned, believes that certain syndromes diagnosed as psychopathic in the USA are due to such early emotional disturbances.

Just as the formation of the ego may be disturbed by partial retardation of development, so also may the development of the super-ego be delayed and hindered. The child's progress will be held back sometimes by insufficient ego development (Guex[52]), at other times by social conditions unfavourable to the formation of his super-ego. Here, it will no longer be a question, as before, of a super-ego normally formed but of antisocial content, but of a super-ego which has not been normally formed. Perhaps the child has lived in unfavourable circumstances and has not had the opportunity to form strong and lasting emotional ties with one or more persons in his immediate circle. Perhaps the child has been morally neglected and has not experienced the necessary emotional forces which will enable him to evolve from the stage of behaviour, where the pleasure and reality principles are finely balanced, to a more-stable and more-highly developed mode of behaviour. The child is hence prevented from completing his moral character and will obey a primitive moral code which, while allowing him to adapt himself to current realities as long as these do not openly clash with instinctive drives, renders him powerless to deal with any serious struggle between these two forces.

This type of case is met with among so-called "badly brought-up" children, whose super-ego is absent because the parents have not been able to exercise that pressure on the child which is indispensable if the energy necessary for super-ego construction is to be set free. Other cases are found among the many children who have been taken away from their families at an early age and have been repeatedly placed and re-placed by the public authorities in a series of foster-homes and institutions, so that they have never had the time or opportunity to achieve firm and lasting emotional relations, necessary to a complete moral development. It is fully to be expected that Bowlby's study [17] will prove scientifically the tremendously important part played by successive changes of abode in the origin of social maladjustment.

Other partial retardations are found in the intellectual sphere: delays in the acquisition of reading and writing (also known as developmental dyslexia) to give but one example which is important both socially and educationally. Space forbids any detailed discussion of this condition, which is more common than is usually believed, and which is the special concern of educational psychologists. I agree with Lauretta Bender (personal communication) that these difficulties can be the starting-point of a feeling of social maladjustment, which in turn, under unfavourable conditions, can become a factor in delinquency. Today diagnostic and therapeutic methods are available which enable the recognition and treatment of these difficulties. It is highly regrettable that educational psychologists should still be prone to underestimate their importance.

I will mention again the point already discussed in the section on organic disease and illness (see page 29), that is the direct, or indirect, influence exerted on the degree of social adaptation by constitutional, and acquired, motor disability, retarded physical growth, sensory infirmities, etc., a mechanism of over-compensation for inferiority feelings being involved.

These partial retardations in development are of varying importance, being sometimes widespread and at others hardly noticeable, or affecting only a small part of the personality. But even then, by means of a kind of psychological law of the " landslide ", they can bring about eventually serious disturbances in mental growth.

2.4.3 *Psychoneuroses and psychoneurotic symptoms*

Although many people today use these terms freely, there is no agreed definition of the concepts they represent. This is a discussion for specialists, and there can be no question of taking part in it here. The following general definition, although pragmatic, must suffice for the purpose of this report: a psychoneurosis consists of a number of pathological symptoms primarily of psychological origin, causally related to each other, exerting a compulsive influence on the behaviour of the patient, and tending to be permanent rather than to remit spontaneously. The classical psychoneuroses are the anxiety neuroses, the obsessional neuroses, and the hysterical neuroses.

It is generally agreed today that these psychoneurotic syndromes are the result of a conflict between the instincts (the " id " of the psycho-analysts), the ego, and the super-ego. These conflicts start in early childhood, the influence of the child's psychological environment interacting with his biological constitution, and can result in the instinctual forces being repressed too little or too much. They may also lead to fixation of certain parts of the personality at earlier stages of development, to partial or extensive regressions to a past level of development, to a pathological displacement of emotional ties from their first object on to others, to the substitution of a poorly adapted and compulsive mode of behaviour for a well adapted and rational one, and to the automatic conversion of one symptom into another.

As well as these fully formed psychoneuroses, many individuals have isolated neurotic symptoms, which have the same origin, and result from the same mechanisms, as the fully fledged psychoneuroses, but which involve the whole personality to a lesser extent, because they affect only certain parts of the individual's emotional and intellectual behaviour and life, and because the individual's ego is sufficiently stable and strong to limit their harmful effects.

For example, such isolated neurotic symptoms may consist of isolated phobias, feelings of inadequacy, states of failure and self-punishment, failure to make good social relations, together with various difficulties with the opposite sex, etc. It is obvious that these are common symptoms. They are present, more or less, in all individuals though it would be an exaggeration to say that we are all psychoneurotics, just as it would be false to say that all those with a positive tuberculin-reaction are tuberculous.

The psychoneuroses and these isolated psychoneurotic symptoms can be distinguished from the simple retardations in development, mentioned earlier by their greater stability, and the slender chances of reversibility and spontaneous cure that they offer.

What correlations are there, therefore, between the psychoneuroses, the isolated psychoneurotic symptoms, and juvenile delinquency?

It is not difficult to understand how some forms of psychoneuroses may predispose to delinquent behaviour. For not only can they, like any other mental illness, result in a severe social " dis-adaptation ", but they can also lead to a kind of compulsive need to commit crimes, as is the case in the obsessional neuroses and indeed in many other neuroses where more subtle mechanisms are involved. This is particularly true of some sexual crimes and also of thefts, fugues, etc. Nevertheless, if reference is made to the definition of psychoneuroses just given, such cases do not seem to me to play an important part in the etiology of juvenile delinquency. In the first place, many psychoneuroses, though originating in early childhood, do not reveal themselves till after puberty. Secondly, while it is true that certain psychoneurotic reactions may favour delinquent behaviour, more often the numerous suppressions and repressions which typify a fully developed psychoneurosis protect the neurotic from his antisocial impulses, which would otherwise make a delinquent of him. Psychoneurotic delinquents exist, beyond all doubt, and are particularly difficult to treat, since they react badly and are recalcitrant to all the usual measures applied to other delinquents. On this score, they warrant special attention, and magistrates and teachers must be aware of all the difficulties they present. Once again, these cases are not numerous, compared to the whole body of juvenile delinquents, and to try to make out that every delinquent is a psychoneurotic is an error which can lead to serious misunderstanding between the psychiatrist, the magistrate, and the re-educator.

On the other hand, isolated neurotic symptoms are often among the most important etiological factors in a juvenile's social " dis-adaptation ". To believe that such factors are effective only where there is a constitutional predisposition to delinquency does not diminish their importance. One of the first tasks of the psychiatrist when collaborating with magistrates and re-educators is to lay bare these symptoms, and explain their mode of action.

Some of these psychological processes will now be considered.

The feeling of being abandoned may at times lead to serious antisocial behaviour through the paradoxical need it produces in children so affected to be for ever re-experiencing the strength of the emotional bonds between them, their parents, their teachers, and society. This need " to test in order to prove ", in Guex's [53] happy phrase, is quite obvious in some of the children who have frequently moved from one home to another, from one institution to another, their behaviour deteriorating " despite " these changes, which a few inexperienced educators believed would be successful. These children's feelings of insecurity are so strong that their antisocial behaviour finally becomes almost compulsive. The need for self-punishment often leads children and adolescents to delinquent acts. The presence of this need can be inferred when the re-educator finds that " gentle methods " fail (which is easily explained since they do not satisfy the child's unconscious need for punishment), whereas " severe methods " seem, at first, completely successful. Soon, however, the child becomes a recidivist, and punishment has less and less effect. Only when the unconscious motives for the wish to be punished are uncovered can the child be helped back to normality. At other times, antisocial behaviour takes the form of agression which may be secondary to anxiety, or primary, when it is the result of a faulty emotional integration, the aggressive instincts not having been amalgamated with the love-forces.[31] The attainment in a symbolic way of repressed wishes may be an important factor in some forms of stealing. Emotional frustration at an oral level is often a cause of taking sweets and other food. A childish desire to share by magic sometimes explains thefts from people admired or loved by the child. Isolated compulsive mechanisms are occasionally found in children who are pyromaniacs, or subject to fugues. This list could be made still longer.

A sound knowledge of these neurotic mechanisms is very necessary and without it the re-educator may make serious and harmful mistakes.

2.4.4 *Psychoses and the psychotic reaction pattern*

It is well known that psychiatrists make a distinction between the " organic " psychoses, the result of macroscopic lesions (senile and arteriosclerotic dementia, general paralysis, post-traumatic dementia, etc.) and the " functional " psychoses, in which, by ways not yet fully understood, the mental functions of the brain are disturbed without its anatomical structure being affected (schizophrenia, manic-depressive psychoses, paranoia, etc.). The organic psychoses will not be enlarged on further here since mention has already been made of those that concern juvenile delinquency in the section on organic disease and illness (see page 29).

Turning to the " functional " psychoses, schizophrenia is the only one of interest here, manic-depressive psychoses being very rare before the age of 18.

Today there is some disagreement amongst psychiatrists over schizophrenia, the concept itself, its symptomatology, incidence, and etiology. While on the one hand the majority of European psychiatrists, together with many American psychiatrists, accept the classic theories of

Bleuler, who described in detail its clinical symptomatology and forms, and traced its etiology to a constitutional and biological origin, on the other hand, a number of psychiatrists and psychologists in the USA appear to extend the concept of schizophrenia well beyond its established boundaries, and give it a psychogenic origin. Thus, Lauretta Bender and her co-workers assert that they have established diagnostic criteria which enable them to diagnose, quite frequently, children aged 2 or 3 as schizophrenics, while psychiatrists of the European school have always considered infantile schizophrenia a rarity. This is not the place to take sides in these discussions, which are referred to here only to explain how the relative importance assigned to schizophrenia in the causation of juvenile delinquency varies from one side of the Atlantic to the other. Without prejudging the issues of the etiology of schizophrenia, its symptomatology, and incidence, it is useful and practical to use the concept of " a psychotic reaction pattern " for want of a better phrase, as one of the possible disorders of mental growth. This phrase would cover a severe personality disorder characterized by chaotic relations between the instincts, the ego, and the super-ego. In this condition, the instinctual forces, no longer controlled or repressed by the ego and the super-ego, break through to the higher levels of the personality, and profoundly disturb the individual's adaptation to reality. Such an illness is quite different from a psychoneurosis, where the personality organization is not completely disrupted, but has become rigid in a conflict for power, ending generally in the strong repression of various instinctual elements.

It is not altogether by chance that the movement to widen the concept of schizophrenia and to give it a psychogenic explanation should take place in the USA. The immigrants who pour into the country in vast numbers each year and, even more, their first generation of children, fall victims of a conflict between the culture of their native countries and the culture of this new civilization to which they must adapt themselves in the pitiless struggle for existence. It is reasonable to believe that such a conflict may lead, in suitably predisposed children, to deep splits in the superego and thereby the door is opened to that degree of chaos which I have called " the psychotic reaction pattern ". It is therefore possible that, although European psychiatrists have difficulty in accepting schizophrenia as a major factor in juvenile delinquency, their American colleagues have many more opportunities for seeing illnesses with symptoms more or less schizophrenic occurring in young people who may be predisposed to this illness.

2.5 Secondary Community Influences: Cinema, Radio, the Press, Alcoholism

The title of this section is taken from a most interesting paper by Clinard [23] which also contains a useful bibliography. I propose to deal quite briefly here with the question of the influence of the press, cinema, radio, organized and unorganized leisure, and alcoholism, on juvenile delinquency.

Once again there is no general agreement on the effects of the press, cinema, and radio, and, in these days, television. The most currently expressed opinion is that all these sensory and emotional stimuli, with their commercialized appeal to the mind, have in varying degrees an important and harmful influence on the general level of morals, especially in young people and children. To give but one example (as quoted by Parker [88]) an examining magistrate remarked " I have not the slightest hesitation in saying that, in my opinion, films and detective thrillers have had, in the vast majority of cases, most harmful effects, and that there is no need to search further for the origin of delinquent behaviour in children and adolescents ". There would be no difficulty in quoting thousands of similar opinions.

If this problem is faced in an objective manner, it will become clear that hardly anything is known for certain about the lasting effects of the cinema, press, and radio on the minds and more particularly the moral growth of young people. To show a film with scenes of violence, or to broadcast a play with an immoral subject, for example, will not be sufficient to arouse the aggressive and antisocial tendencies of a youthful audience. In the first place, for such effect to result, the child must be intellectually capable of understanding what exactly is happening. There is much experimental evidence which shows how children can remain unmoved by scenes which shock their parents, because they do not understand them. In the second place, the child's capacity to live an intense fantasy life must always be taken into account; many experiences lived through on a fantasy level have often little influence on real behaviour, while, in an innocuous manner, a vicarious discharge will have been given to all kinds of antisocial tendencies.

Making use of this hypothesis of the child's reactions to cinema and radio, various authorities have asserted that these amusements not only cause no harm but may have a considerable positive value. Josette Frank, a specialist in the psychology of radio, writes for example (in a quotation by Tappan [125]) " I believe that this type of vicarious adventure, escape, excitement, even blood and thunder is necessary and important to most children as outlets for their own emotions, particularly their feelings of aggression ". In view of present knowledge, such an opinion, though theoretically possible, has as much scientific backing as that of the judge, quoted above. In my opinion, the following points are more or less established, or at any rate, very likely:

(1) These commercialized forms of amusement (cinema, radio, various children's papers, etc.) attract a vast number of children and adolescents in most of the countries of our western civilization. In America, " comics " print at several million copies each, and there are hundreds of such papers

appearing regularly. In France, in 1942, of a total of six million cinema-goers, two million were under twenty. In the USA the corresponding figures are : a total of seventy-seven million weekly cinema-goers, of which twenty-eight million are juveniles (Parker [88]).

(2) Using their own techniques and means of publicity, the cinema, press, and radio occupy a considerable part of the intellectual and emotional life of children and adolescents.

(3) In the present way of life, it is quite clear that, with a few exceptions, these commercialized amusements are not helpful auxiliaries to a child's education or to the growth of his moral sense, any more than they are to his intellectual, aesthetic, and emotional development.

(4) In the light of present knowledge, it cannot be affirmed that these amusements have any specific or major harmful influence on juvenile morality, or on delinquency in particular.

(5) On the other hand, it is well established that the cinema and, to a lesser extent, the radio, can arouse under certain conditions acute anxiety which may, in turn, result in other psychological reactions (aggression, guilt, etc.). Similarly, experience shows that the cinema, radio, and press may teach certain criminal techniques to juveniles predisposed to learn them.

(6) It would seem that the cinema, radio, and press form a group of contemporary, social factors which act by lowering the stability and unity of a community, and by disinhibiting various primitive forms of behaviour.

I find myself, therefore, in agreement with the concluding remarks of a recent article by Lebovici,[74] remarks which are equally true of radio and television : " A film is a reflection of our mental life. In view of its social importance it must have some effect on it. But here is a field where hasty interpretations are particularly rash, and where thorough research is necessary ".

Although this research has not yet reached definite conclusions, it is nevertheless useful to carry on in an objective way, with methods that will remedy ignorance of this most important subject. Important research work is being done at the Institut de Filmologie of the University of Paris, the American Motion Picture Association, New York, the Cinema Research Unit, directed by Ellen Siersted in Copenhagen, etc.

Preconceived opinions are held about the influence not only of the cinema and radio, but also of the free use of leisure, on juvenile behaviour, and on juvenile delinquency in particular. This is certainly a subject that warrants further study. In big towns the free use of leisure is closely linked with the growth of bands of adolescents, those famous " gangs " which seem to play so important a part in juvenile delinquency in the USA.

This problem is not, however, a simple one; that children should spend their leisure in the company of other children may be an excellent training in social adaptation. Care must also be taken not to base assessment of the value of these children's groups on subjective criteria, which may differ profoundly from those of the children themselves.[79] Carroll & Mannheim (personal communication) have undertaken a systematic research programme into this hitherto unexplored subject, and their results will certainly be of use to all criminologists.

Alcoholism has a well established reputation for causing delinquency.

> The alcohol consumed by the juveniles themselves can of course have a harmful result, either through its disinhibiting effect facilitating impulsive delinquent behaviour, or through a permanent deterioration in the higher mental functions, resulting in an increasing social maladjustment. Although there is evidence, here and there, of an increased consumption of alcohol by juveniles, for the time being this does not seem to be a really important factor in juvenile delinquency. Adolescents who regularly drink to excess have nearly always other psychological difficulties, of which alcoholism is but one, though it aggravates the others.

The results of alcoholism in the adults of a juvenile's family circle are quite a different matter. The evil effects of the many mental traumata inflicted on children in their early years by the alcoholism of one, if not both, parents can never be sufficiently stressed. Possibly here, too, alcoholism is but a symptom of an unfavourable psychological predisposition, and is therefore a consequence rather than a primary cause of social degradation. But such a consequence carries with it so many alarming symptoms, and aggravates the situation in which it occurs to such an extent that, from a simple consequence, alcoholism becomes in turn a cause. The social and psychological situation of a family may already be grim, but when alcoholism is added to the picture it becomes dramatic.

Inherited alcoholism is still a subject of debate; once a firmly established dogma, today its influence and very existence is in doubt, particularly since the genealogical studies of the Munich school. It is true that the incidence of intellectual and personality disorders is higher among the descendants of alcoholics than the general population as a whole; but genealogical studies comparing the descendants of an alcoholic with the descendants of his non-alcoholic siblings reveal an almost equal proportion of psychopathological cases in the two groups. On the other hand, the comparison of an unselected group of chronic alcoholics with a group of chronic alcoholics whose medical histories showed that in all probability they had become alcoholics by chance, through force of professional circumstances (commercial travellers, delivery men, etc.) reveals a lower proportion of psychopathological cases amongst the latter group than among the former. These investigations seem to point to the conclusion that what was originally considered to be a specifically alcoholic heredity is in fact but a psychopathic heredity where alcoholism is a complicating factor, or a secondary acquired symptom. Today, therefore, caution must be exercised in the use of the concept of inherited alcoholism, while awaiting the results of further research, which will perhaps finally solve this problem.

2.6 Conclusions — Psychological Common Denominator of Criminal Factors

Throughout this chapter, it has been my aim to describe and to collate current opinions on the main groups of factors which appear to play a part in the etiology of juvenile delinquency. The reader will have noticed the clash of opinions even on those subjects where it should be easy enough to establish the facts, for example the role of mental deficiency. And if, in the section on the disturbances of the psychological development of the personality, I had given a full account of every opinion held on this subject today, my survey would have been even more variegated.

Nevertheless, consideration of all the facts known today leads to the conclusion that delinquency is a "bio-psycho-social phenomenon" in the words of Lafon [71] (in a work in press). No one who wishes to gain an insight into the causes of social maladjustment and of one of its consequences, juvenile delinquency, can afford to neglect any one of the three terms of this expression.

Superficially, everyone seems to be agreed on this point, and further emphasis may therefore appear superfluous. But in fact many people, while seeming open-minded, are found on closer acquaintance to be strongly resistent to new ideas. The deep-rooted nature of these resistances is no doubt partly due to the different disciplines in which the various workers on the problems of delinquency have been trained. Clearly the geneticist in his laboratory, the psychiatrist in his hospital, the sociologist immersed in his statistics, the magistrate in the seat of justice, the re-educator wrestling with human nature, will each have only an incomplete view of one and the same problem. Because their choice of approach reflects their personal, unconscious drives, the re-educator being of a different cast of mind from the sociologist, just as the doctor differs from the magistrate, they will find all the more difficulty in understanding the point of view of a colleague schooled in another discipline.

I have dwelt on these difficulties at some length, because I believe that the medical psychiatrist, apart from his technical functions, can become a most useful link uniting all workers interested in juvenile delinquency. His combined biological and psychological training, his general interest in social problems, his knowledge of the law gained through his medico-legal experience, his understanding of educational problems acquired for personal and professional reasons, will not make him a superman able to solve all problems; but he will have acquired, at any rate, sufficient understanding to attempt to reconcile all points of view, a function for which his training as a psychotherapist specially fits him. I believe that one of the main tasks of the psychiatrist is constantly to emphasize the bio-psycho-social origin of delinquency to all those concerned, and to help them draw the correct conclusions individually, both for a theoretical approach and for research work, and above all to help formulate a practical approach to each worker's daily activities.

This point having been emphasized, it must, however, be remembered that this report is written by a psychiatrist, and the problem of delinquency is approached here from a psychiatric and psychological angle. Does this particular approach permit the discovery of a general principle, or a common denominator of the three facets of juvenile delinquency, biological, psychological, and social?

I believe that this psychological common denominator can be found in the feeling of insecurity to which any criminal tendency from whatever source gives rise. Whether it is a question of a physical illness or infirmity, or an incomplete development of the central nervous system, all such conditions will become obstacles, in one way or another, to the harmonious and complete formation of the ego, which is, as I have shown, the means of adaptation to the necessities of the external social world, and this imperfect adaptation results in objective and subjective insecurity. Whether it is a question of unfavourable social conditions, of financial difficulties, of bad housing, of overcrowding, of harmful and evil companions: or worse, whether it is a question of wars, revolutions, and industrial upheavals: everywhere is found insecurity born of uncertain material and emotional conditions. Whether it is a question of psychological factors, faulty emotional development, instability due to the constitutional components of the personality, overpowering instinctual drives, massive repressions, emotional frustration, feelings of being abandoned, broken family life: in all these are found the psychological conditions engendering insecurity.

It is easy to demonstrate by which psychological processes this insecurity gives rise to anxiety: anxiety, that fear without an object, that apprehension of the unknown to come, little understood even by its victim, but which creates such tension that relief must be obtained at all costs. An aggressive reaction is the most usual method of obtaining this relief, as can be easily proved. This aggressive reaction may sometimes be only slight, but at other times may result in crime, of every variety from the most trivial to the most serious. This criminal behaviour, whether or not it is labelled as such, results in turn in a further reaction, feelings of guilt, at least in those individuals whose moral growth has reached the stage of super-ego formation. But guilt leads to more anxiety, thereby completing the vicious circle—anxiety, aggression, guilt, anxiety. This vicious circle is, without doubt, one of the most constant psychological forces for crime and especially for juvenile delinquency.

CHAPTER 3

PREVENTION OF JUVENILE DELINQUENCY

It is customary in medical treatises to precede the chapter on prevention by one on treatment. I prefer, however, to depart from this rule. For, given the aspect under which juvenile delinquency is considered here, it may be said that a delinquent is a case of social maladjustment whose treatment has either not yet been undertaken or has failed. In other words, the psychiatrist practises the prophylaxis of juvenile delinquency from the angle of the treatment of the psychological disturbances in the social adaptation of young people. The treatment of the delinquent becomes in this way only a special case in the more general treatment of the behavioural disorders of children. I therefore think it is both simpler and more logical to deal with this subject later on. Would it be too optimistic to believe that a day will come when the treatment of the established evil will be replaced by treatment of the threatened disorder, and that the order of importance set up solely by the incompleteness of our medical knowledge will be destroyed ?

In the report of the International Group of Experts on the Prevention of Crime and the Treatment of Offenders, which met at the fifth session of the United Nations Social Commission,[130] the following appears : " Logically, specific preventive measures fall into three categories, viz :

(i) Prevention by early detection and treatment of potential delinquents before they present a manifest problem ;

(ii) Prevention at the stage of pre-delinquency, i.e., by diagnosis and treatment of the " problem personality " ; and

(iii) Prevention of recidivism, i.e., the prevention of the commitment of a crime by persons previously convicted."

The problem outlined in (i) above will constitute the main subject of this chapter whilst those of (ii) and (iii) belong rather to the province of definite treatment.

3.1 General Observations : Aims and Functions of Prophylaxis

What is the object of considering juvenile delinquency and studying the means of its prevention ? The obvious answer is surely that we are seeking to combat adult delinquency with all its train of consequences. Indeed, if juvenile delinquency were a phenomenon strictly limited to persons of less than 18 years of age, without any regard to the future behaviour of the adult, it would scarcely be worth while to devote so much time to its study and prevention. The material harm caused by crimes committed by juveniles is of relatively little importance, and, if the delinquent conduct of boys and girls were merely a kind of youthful measles which could be completely cured, there would be no great cause for anxiety. But it is precisely because of the belief that this malady will have serious and far-reaching consequences that attempts are made to combat it, following the old rule " Principiis obsta ".

On closer consideration the problem is not so simple. The study of concrete facts, notably of the works of such criminologists as S. and E. Glueck, Grassberger, and Frey, reveals that, of the numbers of young delinquents brought before a court, a small percentage only (about 10%-20%) tends to prolong delinquency into adult years. That means that about 80%-90% of the juvenile delinquents brought before a court will not offend again, or at least will not retain their delinquent tendencies beyond the crisis of their juvenile adaptation.

Should then the prophylaxis of delinquency be limited to the 10% or 20% potential adult delinquents ? That is a point to be seriously considered. But there again many questions arise as the problem is more closely scrutinized. First, how can this particularly susceptible fraction be recognized sufficiently early in the general mass of adolescents ? Glueck & Glueck [44] in the USA, and Frey [35] in Europe have made a special study of this question of social prognosis, and they have established criteria whereby it should be possible to foretell the probable evolution of a juvenile towards chronic delinquency. These are indeed investigations of the greatest interest, but they have yet to be tested out on a large scale and their application will probably always present some difficulties and causes of error.

But even if it is admitted that group tests, carried out, let us say, on entering school, may permit the detection at an early age of potential cases of recurring delinquency, the problem would not be solved. For it is not known to what extent these peculiarly susceptible cases will respond to prophylactic measures. It is not unlikely that such cases are victims of very active constitutional factors, which may render all preventive measures undertaken on a re-educational level illusory, or at least very difficult. Again, if success is achieved in keeping them from delinquency in their youth, will that safeguard them later on ? This has not yet been by any means proved, although the general tendency is to accept it as an established fact. Obviously, if the prophylaxis of juvenile delinquency is conceived only from the angle of prevention of adult delinquency, a vast number of problems arise, interesting but so far unsolved, and the whole subject becomes uncertain.

There is, however, another way of considering the prevention of juvenile delinquency. The study of its causes in the preceding section led to the conclusion that, whatever may be the cause of an unlawful act in a minor, this act is the outcome of the vicious circle: insecurity—anxiety—aggression. So that, whether it be a question of an " accidental " juvenile delinquent, who will not become a recidivist, or of a future habitual delinquent, or of any other case between these two extremes, delinquency should appear as a sign: a sign of a passing or permanent, superficial or fundamental, disorder and of a threatened or actual social maladaptation.

Any rational prophylaxis must, therefore, attack the basic disorders of which delinquency is a sign. Its form and scope will be that of a vast mental health campaign: juvenile delinquency will serve as its starting point and raison d'être. A comparison with the modern battle against tuberculosis may illustrate this point. Tuberculosis, like delinquency, is more than a specific malady affecting the individual and society. It is the sign of a physiological, sometimes even of a psychological weakness. Any modern anti-tuberculosis method, serving both as watchword and banner of a hygiene crusade, aims to produce a general improvement in public health and in the individual, family, and social conditions of a community, thereby accomplishing far more than the limited objective of an onslaught on Koch's bacillus.

The battle against juvenile delinquency also appears as the opportunity, unique in its kind, for assembling under a common banner and in a common team-activity public authorities and private agencies, jurists, re-educators; and doctors, specialists and the ordinary public, parents and professional educationalists, theorists and practitioners. It is not unreasonable to expect that from such vast generalized action there should result in time, though doubtless after several generations, a substantial diminution in the number of social misfits hitherto considered as more or less constitutional, and, among them, of habitual or recurrent delinquents. Once again, take the symbol of the soil and its gradual modification by means of the successive contributions of vegetable generations; one has a vision of the way in which human " soils " susceptible to habitual delinquency could also be gradually modified by a patient, systematic campaign.

In this connexion it is interesting to emphasize a fact which cannot fail to strike all those who are concerned with delinquency and psychiatry: I mean the considerable difference which exists in the proportion of the sexes between those appearing at the juvenile courts, those seen at child-guidance centres, and those treated by adult psychiatric outpatient departments. For example, the following are the recorded percentages for Lausanne (Switzerland) over the last three years:

	Juvenile courts		Child-guidance clinics		Psychiatric outpatients	
	F	M	F	M	F	M
1947	18	82	35	65	51	49
1948	17	83	36	64	48	52
1949	14	86	36	64	51	49

F = female   M = male

This table shows that the behaviour considered by society or by the social environment as so antisocial that it calls for penal action, is, grosso modo, five times less in girls than in boys. Does this mean that this lower proportion of delinquency indicates a superior mental equilibrium in the female sex ? Other figures in the table seem to indicate that such an hypothesis would be erroneous. In fact, passing from a consideration of serious social maladjustment, as expressed by the percentage of delinquency, to the milder disorders of mental development, though sufficiently marked to attract the attention of parents and teachers, disorders which are indicated by the proportion of children brought for psychiatric examination to the Office médico-pédagogique vaudois (Switzerland), it is found that the girls are now only half as numerous as the boys. Finally, in the adult clientele of open psychiatric and psychotherapeutic outpatient clinics, where most of the patients come of their own free will because they feel that their mental equilibrium is upset, as many women are found as men. In reality there are even more women than men among patients coming for consultations of their own free will, since the figures here are slightly falsified by the fact that these clinics are obliged to see a certain number of medico-legal or alcoholic cases, a fact which artificially increases the number of male patients. As far as I can judge, similar figures would be found in the statistical returns of similar departments in the USA and Europe.

It seems permissible to give the following interpretation of these facts : if the girls are less delinquent, " better behaved ", more-easily adapted to the exigencies of their surroundings than the boys, it is not because their inner mental equilibrium is better. This is proved by the fact that, once they reach adult age, they are found to have as many and even more psychological disorders whose origin can be traced back to their childhood. But the anomalies of mental development in girls jar less upon society than those of boys. Girls are less aggressive, their difficulties take forms which are considered, wrongly, to be normal feminine traits, and for this reason are more easily tolerated, even accepted with a certain amused and affectionate indulgence : childishness, emotional lability, intellectual inhibitions, a tendency to invent stories about themselves, hysterical behaviour, exaggerated coquettishness, or on the other hand the pose of being " a good little girl ", " as good as gold " " an angel of sweetness " : all examples of behaviour which may be the outcome of neurotic inhibitions. The result is that the little girl's neurosis, developing, as it often does, without any alarming symptoms, goes too long unrecognized. Since it is thus not reached by any therapeutic help, it often leads later to disorders in the mental equilibrium of the adult woman. When this neurotic adult woman becomes a mother, her children will suffer from her difficulties and will present in their time abnormalities in their mental development, and if they are boys they may show manifestly antisocial behaviour, even delinquency. The same process is involved here as in the blood disease known as haemophilia : it is known that it is transmitted through women but is manifest only in men. Treatment of the non-delinquent little girl or teen-age girl might perhaps have been the most efficacious prophylaxis for the delinquency which a few years later will break out in her sons.

Before proceeding now to a brief systematic account, I would like to say something about the American experiment known as the " Cambridge-Somerville Youth Study " whose results, although hitherto no definite publication has been made of them, have already aroused a very lively interest.

The study deals with the observation of two groups of children, 650 boys in all, whose ages at the outset of the experiment ranged from 6 to 12 years. They were divided in equal numbers into an observation group T and a control group C in such a way that, on the basis of the preliminary individual psychological and sociological investigations, it could be agreed that the two groups C and T were composed in as strictly identical a manner as possible, having regard to the age, social environment, intelligence, and character of the 325 children in each. From 1938-1945, group T was studied by a team of social workers : each boy in this group was subject to the constant attention of a social worker; he was helped in his school adaptation, benefited from medical care and organized leisure, and both he and his parents were offered advice on various matters. In short, every effort was made to let the members of group T and their families profit by a well-organized social service inspired by current psychological principles.

Group C on the contrary, being intended to act as a control group, was not under the care of any special social service. In 1948, three years after the close of the experiment which had lasted for eight years, a comparison was made between the groups T and C with special reference to the question of delinquency. No appreciable difference could be found in the frequency of delinquency among the members of group C or group T. (I am deliberately refraining from entering here into too many details and quoting figures for fear of leading the reader to erroneous conclusions based upon a dangerous half-knowledge of the facts.) The first conclusion then in Powers' [95] article, from which I have taken this information, is that the comparison between the number of delinquents in group C and group T, in so far as it is possible to judge after a few years of treatment, proves that " the special work of the counselors was no more effective than the usual forces in the community in preventing boys from committing delinquent acts ".

Such an experiment carried out conscientiously and competently and in as scientific a spirit as is possible to apply to such a problem is disturbing in its result and might make one doubt the value of preventive measures in general. However, the following observations, suggested partly by Sellin, one of the scientific advisers who presided at the drawing-up of the project, and by R. A. Young, one of the leaders of the executive team, should be considered :

(1) The execution of the project was seriously hindered by the war, which caused too many changes in personnel, changes which, it can be readily seen, are particularly regrettable in an experiment where the emotional transference between protected and protectors plays so important a part.

(2) The subjects of the experiment, at the time when they were taken in charge, were all at least six years old (average age 10½). The experiment could thus exercise no influence over the period of early childhood, which, as pointed out in the previous section, is of extreme importance in the genesis of the psychological factors leading to delinquency.

(3) The intention of the initiator of the experiment, R. C. Cabot, was to discover if the methods in daily use by social workers, without the further aid of specialized collaborators, such as psychologists, psychotherapists, and psychiatrists, would be sufficient to prevent delinquency in a given social group. Deliberately, therefore, no attempt was made to apply specialized child-guidance or psychotherapeutic methods to group T. If the experiment leads to the conclusion that group T does not get on any better than group C, one can only conclude, for the moment, that the ordinary methods of social workers are inadequate for the prevention of delinquency. The eventual efficacy of more-specialized methods does not here come into the question.

(4) It would be wise to wait for the future publication of the volume which will give a detailed account of the experiment, its aims, methods, and results. Then, and only then, can a definite judgement of the lessons it contains be expressed.

Without seeking to compare the systematic data furnished by the Cambridge-Somerville study with other figures whose interpretation might call for extensive comment, it is interesting to mention that, whereas in 1930 1,503 Jewish minors were brought before the juvenile court in New York, this figure fell to 256 in 1940. While the increase in juvenile delinquency during the war years shows for the whole of New York City a rate of 60%, the increase among Jewish children was only 20%.[66] Since 1926 the Jewish Board of Guardians has set up not only a remarkable social service organization for the benefit of children and parents, but has also established psychological outpatient departments, facilities for psychotherapy, and excellent inpatient centres. All this is carried out in a bold realistic spirit, and in every case the principles of modern dynamic psychology are applied.[1] The suggestion that this organization has contributed to the remarkable diminution of child delinquency in the Jewish community of New York is very possibly correct.

The etiological factors enumerated in the previous section will now be considered in turn in order to study briefly what can be learnt about the organization of prevention.

Once again it is necessary to remind the reader that this subject is treated only from the psychiatric standpoint and, as with the section on causes, covers only a relatively limited aspect of the problem of prevention.

3.2 Sociological Factors

A Salvation Army officer once summed up the correlation of social and psychological factors in the following admirable sentence : " I have never converted a man with cold feet." In more scientific, through less direct, language it might be said that normal social conditions are the indispensable basis for a child's harmonious psychological development. Many volumes have been written on this subject and many more could be written. I will deal here, and incompletely, only with a few points which appear to offer peculiarly direct correlations with the development of a satisfactory social adaptation.

(1) The importance of the emotional quality of early relations between mother and child should stimulate all sociologists to work for the creation of such social conditions as will enable mothers to remain with their children, at least while they are still small, and prevent their having to work outside the home to supplement the wages of the father. It is well known how serious and often irremediable may be the repercussions on the emotional development of a child who is separated from his mother before the age of three. The system of daytime crèches or nursery schools in which parents can come to see their children every day (which is widespread in the State of Israel) may attenuate the disadvantages caused by the absence of the mother, but it can hardly be proposed as offering a completely

---

[1] A verbal communication from H. Alt, Director-General of the Jewish Board of Guardians, shows that the vast preventive and therapeutic efforts of this society for the last twenty years are mainly due to the direct action of a psychiatrist psycho-analyst, Dr. J. H. W. van Ophuijsen.

satisfactory substitute for the constant presence of the mother in real family surroundings.

(2) Similarly, the possible provision of holidays for mothers of families in the small income groups should be systematically organized. At first glance such holidays may appear to form part of a "luxury" social programme, and be thus of only secondary urgency. In reality, the uninterrupted weight of cares and responsibilities, and accumulated fatigue are often responsible for major mistakes in upbringing by mothers who, were they less harassed, could easily find the strength and perseverance necessary to become good parents.

(3) The influence of housing upon the psychological atmosphere of a family cannot be over-estimated. It is not merely a question of providing hygienic and sufficiently roomy dwellings. Each family group should be provided with sufficient isolation from neighbouring groups. (Many a drama in a child's upbringing is due to neighbours' interfering because a baby cries in the night.) Equally important is the possibility for children to play in the open air somewhere near home, so that the mother-child contact during play, which is so important an educational factor, may be maintained under normal conditions. It would also be highly desirable to care for the aesthetic conditions inside the home even though it may be claimed, often wrongly, that the inhabitants are incapable of appreciating these factors. In reality it is here, in the home, that the prevention of broken families by the desertion of husband, wife, and later of adolescents, should be started.

Among the social experiments in prevention which I have been able to observe at work during my travels in search of information, I would mention the "Chicago Area Project" directed by C. R. Shaw (already mentioned in the previous chapter, page 19). This is an experiment based upon a profound knowledge of the conditions of life and needs of the very poorest districts in an urban population, which are also the most productive of crime, and attempts to base preventive measures upon the direct and active collaboration of those whom they would benefit. Some thirty "groups of neighbours" have been formed in the wretchedest parts of Chicago, and the results seem encouraging. Similar projects exist also in other districts of Chicago and in other towns in the USA, but their guiding principles are more like those of the usual social assistance boards. In Paris, Judge J. Chazal is the patron of an enterprise which makes use of mutual help among young people living in analogous social conditions.

In the Netherlands I was able to obtain information about a new organization, one of its founders, Dr. A. Kaan, Director of the Municipal Service of Social Affairs, in Amsterdam, being kind enough to tell me about it. Here there exists a network of municipal and private societies all judiciously co-ordinated, aiming at the planning of leisure, the organization of teams for games in the public parks of the working-class districts, the formation of character in the years of apprenticeship, the organization of recreational activities for families unable to take a holiday away from town, and so on. This organization is particularly interesting because of its dual character, private and official, the very simple and economical means it uses, and because of its inspiration, which is both social and psychological.

I do not claim to have given an exhaustive list of the interactions of sociology and psychology in the field under study. Such a list would make this report far too long. I have therefore confined myself to making suggestions and have refrained from any attempt at enumerating all that has been done or should be done in this vast, almost untilled, field.

3.3 Somatic and Constitutional Factors

This subsection could be prefaced with the same preliminary remarks made at the beginning of the preceding one. In this extremely wide field, the part played by psychiatry is necessarily limited, but the number of problems which have some psychiatric aspect is very great.

Prevention of constitutional psychopathy as such, if the European conception of this nosological group is accepted, can consist only of eugenic measures. But knowledge of the precise laws governing the hereditary transmission of abnormal personality traits is still too incomplete to justify recommending the submission of certain psychopaths to sterilization. On the other hand, it has often been questioned whether recognized psychopaths should not be prevented from marrying. In Switzerland, Article 91 of the civil code lays down the possibility of such an interdiction. Quite recently the civil and psychiatric authorities in that country discussed whether it would not be well to apply this clause far more widely than has hitherto been the case.

It would seem that the discussions on this question allowed everyone to realize the enormous judicial, social, psychological, and moral difficulties which would follow any widespread interdiction of marriage for psychopaths or the mentally backward. So that, while proposing to be vigilant whenever particular conditions appear to call for the application of the Article in question, Swiss public authorities and psychiatrists seem for the moment to have given up the idea of having recourse to new legislative measures which would reinforce the status quo.[10, 11]

In the case of psychopathic personalities, if the opinions advocated in the USA, notably by Lauretta Bender, are accepted, a real causal prophylaxis of this condition would be possible by ensuring the harmonious development of the child before the age of five.

If the hypotheses, for which there is now good evidence, on the importance of intrauterine disease and physical traumata at birth for the future mental development can be verified (see page 24) there will be new possibilities for the prophylaxis of psychopathy, which need not be discussed here.

But, practically speaking, the problem is not so much the prevention of a psychopathic predisposition itself, but rather the prevention of its manifestations in any one individual under any one set of circumstances. In this connexion more suitable measures are available, which give rise to far fewer scientific, social, psychological, moral, or deontological objections, than the strictly eugenic measures just mentioned.

The first thing to do is to help the psychopath to manage his shortcomings, even to benefit by them if that be possible, and not to be a source of worry to his fellow beings on account of them. This end can often be accomplished by the early application of re-educational methods,[g] by intelligent vocational guidance, and by understanding action in connexion with parents and surroundings. In acute cases, or when the home conditions are unfavourable, placing the child in a special institution or in a carefully chosen foster family may result in a relatively satisfactory re-adaptation to the demands of society. Generally speaking—and I shall come back to this point—I do not consider that removal of a child from his family should be too easily resorted to. Certain psychopaths probably provide one of the least contestable indications for such a measure. Once he has reached the post-puberty stage, the psychopath can often benefit from being incorporated in some youth organization, since he finds in a relatively numerous society more possibilities for adaptation than in the restricted circle of family or small work community (but the great variety of psychopaths must be taken into account and there are some for whom the contrary is true).

The child-guidance clinics [h] are organizations specially suited to dealing with the definitely psychiatric aspect, and often with the social and educational aspect, of such cases.

In a more general way, the mental health section of the municipal health services of Amsterdam (which, for a population of some 800,000 inhabitants employs 15 psychiatrists and 15 specialized social workers) is a remarkable example of what can be done towards the socialization of the highest possible number of psychopathic personalities.

It is well known that those forms of mental deficiency which might play a part as etiological factors in delinquency are pre-eminently hereditary in character (the various forms of gross imbecility and idiocy, which are not so often inherited, play in fact only a subordinate part in delinquency). If it should be proved that mental deficiency is a factor leading to delinquency, eugenic measures taken with feeble-minded parents should offer an efficacious prophylaxis for delinquency.

Putting aside, however, the general problems arising from such measures, to which I referred just now, it is not really certain (as has been seen) that mental deficiency is an important factor in producing juvenile delinquency. This scientific uncertainty indicates the necessity for extreme

---

[g] In Holland and the Scandinavian countries there are special schools for psychopaths of normal intelligence.

[h] The term " child-guidance clinics " is here used to designate child psychiatric outpatient departments in their various forms including the child-guidance clinics in England and the USA.

caution in intervention, whether it be a question of sterilization or of prevention of marriage. At all events, the illusion should not be cherished that thereby a really important advance in the diminution of juvenile delinquency is being accomplished. It may be that the future will provide fresh and more precise information on this subject.

For the moment, one thing appears certain : by allowing mentally defective children to benefit by training and teaching appropriate to their limited powers, by preventing in them, and in their parents, the growth of inferiority feelings which all too often develop into aggressivity, one can in many cases avoid there being added to this intellectual weakness those behavioural difficulties which may transform simple mental defectives into antisocial and even criminal defectives. Every child psychiatrist knows that a carefully guided mental defective, provided he is not a morbidly over-active type, can become a harmless, albeit deficient, member of a society, which accepts him for what he is and loves him as he is. On the other hand, the embittered defective, who meets the affronts, to which he is constantly subjected, with force or cunning, may become a dangerous malefactor and difficult to correct. Reference has already been made to Ramer's study [98] from which it would appear that the former pupils of the classes for backward children in Stockholm do not become delinquents in numbers above the overall average for the youths of this city, a fact which seems to prove the usefulness of such specialized teaching.

The attitude of parents, and of society in general, towards mental defectives is very deep-rooted. Gradually intellectual achievement has been put on a pedestal, in the same way as modern society worships money and material success. The re-establishment of a healthier hierarchy of mental values, wherein intelligence would once again take its proper place as a tool in the service of higher values, is a task which may be outside the province of mental health, yet is very directly concerned with it.

The prevention of those organic diseases and illnesses which may have an influence upon delinquency (see page 29) is not a task for psychiatry, which is, however, concerned with the prophylaxis of the psychological consequences which these diseases or illnesses may bring about.

It has already been pointed out how these consequences may consist of inadequate compensation for inferiority feelings in a frequently aggressive form. Encouragement of a sick or crippled child, helping him to find the right adaptation to his particular situation, aiding his parents in a task they often find extremely difficult, constitute an important part of the prevention of maladjustment. Experiments with war-wounded children have shown on the one hand how violent may be the aggressive outbursts of such children, and on the other hand their extreme adaptability if they can be given appropriate orthopaedic treatment, and above all comprehensive psychological guidance.

Societies for helping cripples, specialists in vocational guidance, orthopaedic specialists, and generally speaking all those who deal with crippled children, have an important task to perform here, but which can be brought to fruition only by the use of certain basic psychological knowledge which is often lacking.

Long periods in hospital may also result in disastrous consequences for social adaptation. Diabetic children, tuberculous children, and many others suffering from chronic illnesses which necessitate their being kept for a long time in the all too permissive, yet frustrating, atmosphere of hospitals and sanatoria, may gradually become markedly antisocial, and it may be very difficult once they are physically cured or stabilized to restore them to a satisfactory social adaptation. What a paradoxical and heart-breaking result of the perfecting of medical technique is this division in the care given to the health of the body which can bring about that — I have a concrete case in mind — a child saved by a miracle of surgical skill after years of battling against a tenacious infection can become, a few years later, a practically incorrigible and hardened criminal.

But there is another aspect the importance of which is only beginning to be perceived thanks, among others, to the work of Spitz,[120,121] to which the work by Bowlby,[17] will doubtless make important fresh contributions: the far-reaching consequences of prolonged periods in hospital on quite small children. Owing to a rigorous application of asepsis and dietetics, paediatricians have gained over infant mortality one of the most glorious and triumphant victories in all the history of medicine. But a series of facts compels us to ask ourselves very seriously today whether we have not travelled too far along this victorious path, and whether in particular bacteriological asepsis has not been practised to the advantage of what might be called " mental anaemia ". The systematic exclusion of parents from most of the hospital wards for babies, the standardization of treatment, in particular of feeding, leading to the suppression of many emotional factors in the relations between the baby and its surroundings, would seem to be capable of producing, in a certain number of cases at least, disorders in later social adaptation which are not easily reversible. In the USA, many paediatricians are now revising their methods which only a few years ago seemed part of the most firmly established tenets in child medicine. In Europe, Professor R. Debré of Paris defends the same principles, and similar tendencies are to be found in the University Paediatric Clinic of the Rigshospital of Copenhagen under the direction of Professor P. Plum. It would be of the greatest interest to elucidate definitely and as rapidly as possible the part played by these factors. If they are really as important as present knowledge allows us to believe, it will be necessary, in order to convince the paediatricians, to present irrefutable arguments, for only then will they consent to abandon methods which from a purely physical point of view have given such apparently brilliant results.

3.4 Disturbances in the Psychological Development of the Personality

Educational and social rather than psychiatric measures are involved in the avoidance of formation of an antisocial super-ego and it is unnecessary to dwell at length upon the influence immoral parents may have upon their children. Psychiatry can, however, be consulted on the subject of the proper measures to be taken to protect children against the dangers threatening them. Psychotherapy will be generally ineffective, since it is not a question of removing pathological mechanisms but of substituting one moral ideal for another. In most cases it is necessary to take the child away from its surroundings. In certain cases it will be enough to institute active individual guidance allowing the child to establish new emotional bonds with healthy people; this will constitute the basis for the future modification of his super-ego.

The disorders grouped together in the preceding chapter under the heading " Partial retardation in development " (see page 32) offer on the other hand many opportunities for psychiatry. In connexion with the possible consequences of babies' prolonged stay in hospitals, the probable effects of early emotional frustration on the later development of personality have been once again pointed out in the preceding paragraph. It is obvious that separation in a crèche or hospital is not the only occasion on which such frustrations occur. The inner attitude of mind in which a mother waits for and then receives her baby, the anxiety caused by maternity, the feelings she experiences towards her child, the psychological role of the new-born baby in the life of the mother or of both parents — spoil-sport, obstacle to a proposed divorce, result of an involuntary " accident " and so on — disappointment or resentment in the mother when faced with certain behaviour or certain characteristics in the baby, who perhaps is not of the desired sex, or looks too much like the family-in-law, cries too much, eats badly, does not smile, and so on, all these things, and many other similar psychologically imponderable factors, may prevent the mother from lavishing upon her child that spontaneous, natural, and unwavering affection which is as important a food for the baby's soul as milk is for its body. But still other causes may arise to disturb the harmonious relations between mother and baby : feeding or training principles too rigorously adhered to, uncertainty arising from ill-digested psychological reading or lectures — a phenomenon which seemed to me relatively frequent in the USA — and then again, of course, a series of weightier and more serious causes : difficulties arising through the coming of younger brothers and sisters, neurotic mothers, parents deliberately taking no interest in their children, conjugal dissension leading to separation or divorce : all these causes (and many more could be added) can contribute singly or together to depriving the child of that atmosphere of emotional security which is indispensable to the smooth development of his ego.

The formation of the super-ego depends also to a large extent upon the nature of family relations : as between the father and mother on the one hand and between parents and child on the other. It may be said, as a general rule, that all factors tending in one way or another, directly or indirectly, to diminish the specifically feminine traits in the mother and the specifically masculine traits in the father will set up difficulties in the formation of the superego. In the same way, factors which prevent the child, towards the age of four or five, from forming strong emotional ties with persons who could serve as a model adapted to his sex and stage of development, will delay the moment when the important bridge between infancy and school-age is crossed. Each of these difficulties can give rise to permanent forces for social maladjustment which may in their turn entail the risk of delinquency.

It is interesting to note, in this connexion, that the Chinese colony of San Francisco has a very low percentage of juvenile delinquency. A social worker employed in the Chinese quarter of this town told me that the Chinese in San Francisco, who number some 25,000, continue to lead a social life in the USA very similar to that of their compatriots who remain in their own country. From the educational point of view three facts should be noted : first, the family setting remains very strong and stable, and is based on a hierarchy; secondly, the Chinese family comprises not only parents and children, but various grandparents, uncles, aunts, and cousins, so that the family group may frequently consist of 30 or 40 persons; thirdly, the attitude of Chinese mothers to their babies is extremely tolerant and affectionate. They are separated as little as possible, they take their babies with them if they go out to work, comfort them when they cry, and suckle them whenever the baby makes his demand. Towards the age of five, the mothers' attitude changes, the child is encouraged to behave more independently, more like a grown woman if it is a girl, and more like a man if it is a boy. It would be rash to affirm without further proof that there is a correlation of cause and effect between the low percentage of juvenile delinquency and the cultural pattern of this Chinese community. It is, however, impossible not to be struck by the fact that in these communities conditions prevail which correspond exactly to the theoretical postulates of depth psychology.

This enumeration of possible causes of early disorders in the formation of ego or super-ego contains in itself, without much need for emphasis, an indication of the prophylactic measures which could be applied on a large scale; preparation of the parents, especially of the mother, before the birth of the first child, providing them with advisers on all the problems of growing up which may arise during the early months and years of their children's lives; dealing, in a general way, with the psychological disorders, even though slight, which may affect the parents; the prevention of conjugal conflicts : such is the mental health work which seems to be directly related to the prevention of delinquency.

It is well to remember that simple advice given to parents, though far from useless, is rarely sufficient. Emotional reasons prevent certain mothers from ordering their behaviour in conformity with advice which, nevertheless, on the intellectual plane, they recognize as judicious. It is, therefore, necessary that child-guidance workers, psychologists, and psychotherapists should reach the deeper emotional levels of the parents' personal problems and should bring about, in one way or another, those displacements and re-adjustments without which the advice they give will never penetrate further than the surface, and, for example in a mother who is equally convinced of the wisdom of the advice offered and of her own incapability to follow it, may even create distress, which is far more harmful than the errors it sought to correct. Great Britain leads the way with some interesting experiments in this field.[67]

In the USA I should like to call attention to (among others) the Rochester Child Health Institute, an experiment of wide scope, carried out in collaboration with the Mayo Clinic, initiated by Dr. H. E. Helmholz and now directed by Dr. B. Spock. This is a medico-social organization which, in a spirit of research and prevention, aims at following up all the children in Rochester, Minnesota, born after 1 January 1944, in as thorough a manner as possible, taking into account both the physical and psychological aspects of the child's personality, together with his home and school difficulties, and so on.

I have dwelt particularly upon measures applicable to young children because I share the views of those modern authors who trace back to this period of a child's life the origin of the tendency to most social " disadaptation ", even if it is manifest only much later on. It would therefore seem right to bring the chief prophylactic efforts to bear upon early childhood. But it would be a great mistake to neglect adolescence and school-age. The soil prepared in early life, however favourable it may be to the growth of tiresome weeds, can nevertheless often be cleared, or the growth prevented by later intervention. And again, in certain cases which are most liable to become delinquent, such a soil is of very slow formation ; in these cases personality growth is retarded, and judicious action taken while the child is at school, or even in some cases during adolescence, may have a decisive effect upon the delayed completion of their ego or super-ego.

Important though it undoubtedly is, I do not think one should exaggerate the part played by the school in the genesis or in the prevention and treatment of social maladjustment. It is, however, very desirable that teachers and school authorities should be acquainted with the modern data of the psychology of the child's emotional development and that they should endeavour to organize the school programmes and methods in the light of this knowledge, and above all try to make their daily personal actions conform to the teachings of this psychology when they are with their pupils.[13]

After school-age, adolescence presents peculiarly difficult problems, all the more so since this period of " revolt against conditioned reflexes " as the Swiss psychiatrist, Klaesi, calls it, is relatively ill-understood. Reference on this subject should be made to the works of Debesse of Strasbourg and his development of the science he proposes to call " hébélogie ".

It would take the reader too far if I were to enter into all the details concerning methods of action applicable to school-age and adolescence. Moreover in principle this action is analogous to that just described, though adapted to older subjects. Extra-family organizations, youth clubs, boy scouts or girl guides, religious or political societies specially designed for young people, can all exercise a beneficial social influence on antisocial tendencies. It is during this period that certain aggressive tendencies (often camouflaged) appear in various forms and may lead to the first crime, such as larceny or petty theft. Parents and teachers should be on the alert for possible symptoms of such aggressivity and react accordingly. The reader should consult, for a more complete study of the different aspects of this problem, the work of the International Conference on Child Psychiatry held in London in 1948.[97]

The prevention of the occurrence of psychoneuroses and other psychoneurotic traits capable of leading to juvenile delinquency is a formidable task calling for general mental health, and particular psychotherapeutic measures, and needing very specialized techniques.

It would be tedious to state here the rules of mental health calculated to prevent the growth of neurotic conditions in children. Everyone knows the requirements of psychiatrists, psychologists, and re-educators in this connexion. Moreover, some of them were mentioned when speaking of partially retarded development. To explain the various psychotherapeutic techniques used with neurotic children or adolescents would be to go far beyond the scope of this report. Let me then merely emphasize the importance of all these measures and mention only a few particular points.

As regards general prevention, it seems necessary to remind the public that it is not enough to write pamphlets or organize lectures on educational subjects, although such things have their uses. Propaganda for a better mental health system should be as direct and concrete as possible. The personality of those affected must be reached through their own emotions and problems, so as to arouse a realization of their need for enlightenment and guidance. Small discussion groups organized for parents, and short plays setting forth some problem of the daily emotional life followed by organized discussions [i] are particularly appropriate means of spreading efficiently and incisively modern psychological and educational principles. Parents' associations, private or official organizations for the use of leisure, the organization of holidays, people's universities, all kinds of social services, recreational communities, cinema clubs, etc., all provide means for effective action in favour of better health, provided that really qualified personnel are available for this work. One of the pitfalls to be avoided

---

[i] The American Theatre Wing, Inc., New York, is doing highly interesting work in this connexion.

in such work is to bring to the surface difficulties which are then only partially solved, and thus create in the minds of those approached more insecurity, disorder, and anxiety, than enlightenment and peace of mind. With regard to the psychotherapeutic techniques used with children who are in any way neurotic, it is of the utmost importance that they should be practised only by persons who are very well qualified for this kind of work. Methods may vary; the main thing is that the person who uses them should know exactly what he is doing and what he is aiming at, and should be master of his technique. It must, however, be recognized that any method which takes no account of the knowledge now available of the child's unconscious life, the laws governing the development of his instincts, his emotional life, or his intelligence, and the structure, dynamics, and economy of his mental life, must be considered as definitely out of date.

If one believes (and, as I have said, not everyone is of this opinion) that the psychoses and a particular structural fault in the personality, corresponding to what I have called the " psychotic reaction pattern ", play a part in juvenile delinquency, it must be recognized that the prevention of such states still appears extremely problematic. On the one hand, the constitutional biological element in such illnesses is probably particularly pronounced and offers little opportunity for the exercise of psychological measures. The only logical prophylactic action would be eugenic. The objections that can be maintained with regard to such methods have already been set forth. On the other hand, there is as yet very little information about the first signs of growth of a psychosis in a child. It is quite possible that certain symptoms may exist in a child's behaviour which would give warning of the later development—most frequently after puberty—for example of schizophrenia. But too little is still known for such symptoms to be detected with any certainty and for the prophylactic action to be undertaken which knowledge thereof would indicate. The furnishing of objective and precise anamnestic information, which will perhaps enable, in the relatively near future, the revealing with certainty of the first roots of a psychosis at an early age, is far from being the least useful result of the numerous observations carried out today by child-guidance clinics.

The hypothesis formulated concerning the possible genesis of certain psychotic traits arising from a conflict in the formation of the super-ego may also furnish some prophylactic indications.

Finally, mention should be made of the work carried on for several years now by Lauretta Bender in her clinic at the Belle Vue Hospital, New York, where she not only believes she can diagnose cases of schizophrenia in children at the age of three, but also gives such cases shock-treatment with results she considers to be encouraging.

3.5 Secondary Community Influences: Cinema, Radio, the Press, Alcoholism

I will treat this subject very briefly. On the one hand, as has been pointed out, what is known about the effect of these factors, apart from alcoholism, is still somewhat vague. On the other hand, practical action in this field is certainly outside the province of psychiatry. Psychiatrists and psychologists have, however, an important contribution to make to the study and solution of the problems arising here. Not only can they explain the action of certain factors in the light of their own special knowledge (for instance the psychological laws relating to the cinema, radio, or press), but they can also contribute the results of their observations and practical experience of the harmful effects of any one factor on the mental life of children and adolescents.

Actually it is the cinema particularly which presents today the most acute and most difficult problems to solve. (Although already the influence of television is, quite rightly, disturbing some re-educators.) I will not revert to what I have already said about what is known of its influence, nor the importance of the studies to be pursued in this connexion. From the prophylactic point of view the question is whether present knowledge is sufficient to warrant certain measures such as the selection of special films for children, the fixing of a minimum age for admission to certain plays, and the application of precise criteria in the censoring of films. Everyone agrees that something must be done. Opinions vary chiefly on the methods to be employed. Legislation generally appears too cautious : it is, perhaps, feared that too strict an opposition to the extraordinarily powerful attraction of the cinema to adolescents, and even children, may cause general discontent and encourage deception. Public authorities are generally content to give moral support to voluntary efforts, which aim either at selecting special films for children, or developing the taste of parents and children for good pictures or plays. Considering the powerful influence of the cinema through propaganda, good or bad, the efficacy of such efforts may be doubted. Children's cinema clubs such as exist in England[j] are an interesting experiment, though one may wonder whether in the end they do not help the child to develop the habit of, or even the need for, continually going to a picture theatre.

The government of the Canton of Vaud, Switzerland, deliberately choosing a different line of approach, has just published a new decree on the cinema. This not only defines the functions of the film control commission, but in principle forbids the admission to a cinema of any child under seven years of age. Juveniles of 7 to 16 are admitted only to certain films passed by a special commission on children's films. Finally, the film control commission may propose that the minimum age for admission to a particular film should be raised from 16 to 18. The provisions of this decree are, as far as I know, the most up-to-date in this connexion, and they will doubtless furnish material for some interesting experiments.

As regards the factor of alcoholism, the problem of prophylaxis is vast; lack of space prevents any exposition of its data and technique. Many works have dealt with this matter. In view of the so-called medical arguments which are obstinately and often insidiously spread by those with an interest in alcohol who find for this purpose very obliging agents even among doctors, I wish once again to emphasize the gravity of the danger of alcoholism and the urgent need for combating this most pernicious mode of social intoxication.

3.6 Conclusions

By the end of this chapter it may be thought that the subject has been treated too widely, depth having been sacrificed to breadth, that too many

---

[j] For example, the " Children's Entertainment Films " under the patronage of the Rank Organization, but with an independent directing council.

aspects have been considered and no useful conclusion reached, too many questions asked, and few satisfactorily answered. But the aim here was precisely to show the complexity of the tasks involved in prophylaxis, and the foolishness of seeking a panacea in view of the variety of etiological factors and the number of contacts between recurrent or occasional juvenile delinquency and law, sociology, education, and mental health; on the contrary, as long as what is known on the subject remains vague only a multidimensional conception of delinquency and its prophylaxis can lead to some measure of success.

The aim of this intentionally broad and varied study has been to assign their proper place to the tasks of psychiatry and the psychiatrist. I hope I have shown that modern psychiatry cannot be confined to control of antisocial manifestations as related only to the recognized forms of mental disease, such as obvious mental defect, serious psychopathy, or acute psychoneurosis. Of course these conditions will always be of central importance in psychiatry and constitute its most specific field of action. Any psychiatrist not knowing or neglecting them runs the risk of rapidly becoming vague and speculative, and losing the basic qualities of a medical discipline. Nevertheless modern psychiatry has its place outside these restricted boundaries, whenever it is necessary to study, or to influence, the way a person reacts, with his whole personality, to a given circumstance, whether it be a material event, a social fact, or a personal problem. Recalling B. Glueck's aphorism quoted earlier (see page 20), I would say that the general task of psychiatry is to study how a given factor may act upon an individual to produce psychological reactions turning this factor into a force that is felt, thought, and integrated in his personality, to become the final or effective cause of a given behaviour; and the study completed, to use it as the basis of therapeutic and prophylactic action.

With regard to the role of the psychiatrist, he too will not confine himself to the diagnostic, prophylactic, or therapeutic techniques of his own speciality. Using his psychological knowledge and his human interest to understand the social interrelations about him, he will strive to become an instrument for mutual understanding between the various groups concerned with juvenile delinquency: primarily between parents and children, but also between children and re-educators, between re-educators and parents, between the different social workers, between magistrates, educators and doctors, and between delinquents and society. One of the most effective means of such psychiatric collaboration is furnished by the work of the child-guidance teams now found almost everywhere in Europe and the USA, and comprising medical specialists and psychologists and social workers trained in diagnostic and therapeutic work. These teams, owing to their flexibility and the singleness of aim of the many collaborators, can be employed on every front in mental health;

from individual consultations given to parents who spontaneously ask for help, to official specialized reports on given cases of delinquency; from public lectures on mental health subjects to small discussion groups where parents endeavour to analyse emotional problems; from individual treatment of a particular delinquent to regular conferences with the staff of reform institutions; from advice given to re-educators to playing an active part in formulating the laws and regulations concerning the mental health of children; from technical training for staff of reform institutions to university lecturing; in fact, wherever child guidance can be of service. Child guidance is an indispensable weapon in the up-to-date equipment of any community which hopes to wage war successfully against juvenile delinquency and against all forms of social maladjustment.

CHAPTER 4

TREATMENT OF JUVENILE DELINQUENCY

Following this full discussion of the prevention of juvenile delinquency, there is relatively little to say about its treatment, since this includes various technical aspects beyond the scope of this report, and since the contribution of psychiatry is smaller here than in the field of prevention.

4.1 "Primum non Nocere"

This old medical proverb should be observed by all those who apply, whether personally or by proxy, corrective or re-educative measures to young offenders. As was shown at the beginning of this report, the term juvenile delinquents includes many varied and dissimilar types and it was also emphasized that a great number of juveniles, classed as delinquents by the law, do not in fact show any very different psychological traits from other " normal " young people and should not therefore be thought of as pathological cases. These young offenders have the best social prognosis and will often take their place in society as normal, stable individuals, after one single criminal act or brief delinquent period. It should not be forgotten that the very fact of being labelled " delinquent " can set in motion specific psychological reactions even in a youth with no abnormalities in his psychological make-up, whose crime is due primarily to social and accidental causes. In other words, the fact alone of some action being taken about him may profoundly affect his mental outlook. To have a psychological effect on the delinquent is, doubtless, the purpose of such action. It follows, then, that those who decide on such measures shoulder a grave responsibility as to the final result of their decision. Will the good results of re-education and therapy outweigh the harmful effects: resentment, feelings of lowered self-respect, undesirable contacts, and the unleashing of reactive aggression ? As was mentioned at the beginning of the report, it is often extremely difficult to answer this question in advance; the seriousness of the measures suggested or carried out often far exceeds practical or theoretical knowledge which should give us a solid foundation on which to base such measures. The purposive disruption of the family, the openly declared war by the judicial and administrative authorities on the delinquent's family, his dispatch to a corrective centre whether for treatment or prolonged observation, are steps of the utmost gravity, which social workers, be they magistrates, municipal officers, or doctors, have employed with too little thought, perhaps, at times. Naturally, there are occasions when such steps are necessary. Nevertheless, the extreme seriousness, indeed the awful gravity, of such steps must always be borne in mind, since they may be decisive events for good or ill in a delinquent's life.

My investigations in Europe and America revealed that follow-up studies of the work of re-educational centres are both rare and inconclusive. This state of affairs has many causes and it is no easy matter to plan a detailed and penetrating scientific investigation. Nevertheless, one feels uneasy on hearing the variety of suggestions made on re-educative methods, their duration, their timing and technique of application, at a congress of specialists and technicians, with each speaker confidently giving his opinion, often without being able to base it on solid and objective evidence such as would thoroughly convince his audience. The psychiatrist is trained to seek out the psychological sequence of cause and effect; he has observed many times the long-term and serious effect of events which initially seemed of little importance; he knows the paradoxical behaviour of human beings, the concentrated aggression hidden behind a meek exterior, or the deep despair masked by apparent revolt. His role, therefore, is to urge all whose difficult task involves applying corrective measures, to adopt a respectful and cautious attitude towards others, and to youth in particular. This paucity of knowledge should in no way prevent the pursuit in each case of all the necessary investigations which will throw light on the delinquent's personality, on the fundamental motives for his behaviour, and on the best measures for his social rehabilitation. In other words any decision must be fortified by a diagnosis, itself based on a clinical examination.

4.2 Clinical Examination

It should hardly be necessary today to insist on the need in juvenile delinquency for clinical examination and diagnosis. All that has been said on the multiplicity of possible etiological factors irrefutably shows that, far from being satisfied with the simple fact that a youth is delinquent, on the contrary, the fundamental motives of his behaviour must be sought. An "accidental" delinquent, the victim of social forces, needs to be treated in a very different way from another delinquent who is psychologically seriously disordered. And again, within the group of the psychologically disordered, the adolescent whose antisocial behaviour is due purely and simply to the absence of a super-ego should be dealt with differently from the adolescent whose thefts are part of an obsessional psychoneurosis. The correct treatment for the one would drive the other into further delinquent behaviour.

Such views as these, though they seem obvious, still meet in practice with stubborn and perhaps unconscious resistances especially among re-educators. Elsewhere I have set out [12, 13] the reasons for this attitude, and how the born teacher dislikes probing his pupil's past record, preferring to look to the future. Despite the sympathy which activates this attitude, sometimes with good results, it cannot be recommended as an example for others to follow. On the contrary, the medical and psychiatric method of careful family- and personal-history taking and of elucidating the psychological sequence of criminal factors is today considered essential, the value of this method being not at all diminished by the occasional successes of educationalists endowed with brilliant intuition. Any decision taken about a delinquent youth, should, as a matter of principle, be preceded both by a clinical examination and diagnosis.[k]

In practice, in the majority of cases, this need not take up a great deal of time, and could take place quite naturally within the framework of the usual investigation and could be undertaken by magistrates or officials, neither medically nor psychologically qualified, but who are sufficiently experienced and show an enlightened interest in psychological problems.

There may well be some psychiatrists who disagree with this suggestion, but it is necessary to be realistic. To require that each and every delinquent shall be examined by a psychiatrist or specially trained psychologist is a demand impossible to fulfil at present, unless the psychiatric examination is to become a mere formality which would entail far more disadvantages than advantages.

Having conceded this much to common sense and the realities of the situation, there is more justification in suggesting that a medical and psychological opinion must be sought whenever there is the slightest doubt about the genesis of the delinquent's behaviour, though the magistrate, in making the final decision, is free to accept or reject this opinion.

In a recent study, my colleague, Dr. J. Bergier [7] has discerningly defined the scope, requirements, and conditions of outpatient and of inpatient psychiatry. He sums up the advantages of outpatient psychiatry, as follows:

(1) it saves time and money;

(2) it saves the youth losing a good job and cutting short his apprenticeship;

(3) only cases likely to benefit or where there are no contra-indications are sent to rehabilitation centres or to inpatient observation units;

(4) it makes for good relations between patient and doctor, the latter being then considered an ally, rather than a part of the legal system, as happens when the doctor is seen for the first time in the setting of an institution. Moreover, contact with the accused's family becomes both easier and more useful.

---

[k] Aichhorn, who was recognized by all who knew him as a remarkably intuitive and extraordinarily brilliant teacher, always liked to stress how much he owed to his scientific knowledge of psychology, a point fully borne out by his work.

(5) Finally, if psychotherapy is considered necessary on clinical examination, there is less difficulty in initiating treatment when the first contact with the doctor has been in the calmer atmosphere of the consulting-room, rather than in an impersonal office, often felt to be hostile, of an institution or observation centre.

Bergier also draws attention to the dangers of preventive detention, and suggests that a youth should have a short psychiatric examination before the magistrate in charge decides to send him away for observation in an institution. Despite the many technical problems which require solution, this plan will surely meet with approval, particularly in those countries, still numerous, where there are no institutions devoted to the observation of delinquents and where clinical examinations are necessarily carried out, and the diagnosis made, in the setting of a reform school. But even when such special observation centres exist, the type of case sent there must be carefully chosen. Some of the centres, both in Europe and in America, lack the organization to ensure that their inmates do not do themselves more harm than good.

The child-guidance clinics already frequently mentioned in this report are well suited to provide this outpatient psychiatry if they are supplied with the correct technical equipment.

If this brief, preliminary outpatient examination shows institutional observation to be desirable or necessary, it must be possible to send the case to a special institution. As a general rule I am firmly against sending delinquents for observation to a centre devoted to rehabilitation, though an ever-decreasing number of re-educators may disagree. Not only is this practice harmful to the delinquent himself, but it also seriously dislocates the normal routine of the centre, where one should be able to work in an atmosphere of stability and continuity, without the disturbing comings and goings of cases under observation.

> There are several types of observation centres and it must be admitted that the ideal is yet to be found. With so many different cases under its care an institution must take a number of safety precautions, though at the risk of their becoming like prisons. To find the happy medium requires highly gifted re-educators, and the help of a large and well-trained staff. That the problem can be satisfactorily solved is shown by Youth House, New York, and other successful experiments. Furthermore, it is useful to have a number of relatively small centres each with their own methods.

The great difficulty of observation centres lies in reconciling the needs of objective observation with the re-educative work, which inevitably begins in the very first hour a juvenile delinquent spends in an institution. Ideally, of course, observation should have nothing to do with re-education, and should be limited to recording a juvenile's behaviour and his spontaneous or induced reactions. But in practice, this ideal is impossible to realize completely. A transference relationship is bound to arise between the juvenile delinquent and the adult staff around him, and from then on their behaviour will influence him, and thus re-educate him, whether it is desired or not. Besides, it must be remembered that the first days without freedom, often causing an emotional shock, are very favourable to re-education. It is a great mistake to lose this opportunity by leaving the delinquent languishing in a cell or by adopting too diagnostic an attitude. But the staff of these observation centres must avoid the opposite mistake of taking advantage of their charges' misery at being abandoned to set up massive transference and counter transference, which make only more difficult the juvenile's later re-adaptation to his home or hospital, the real settings of his re-education.

It is clear that a satisfactory solution of this problem is yet to be found and that the perfecting of the techniques to be used in these centres requires the co-operation of magistrates, teachers, and psychiatrists.

4.3 Outpatient Treatment

Provided the necessary technical resources are available, the outpatient treatment of juvenile delinquents will often meet with success and be economical, while also avoiding the disadvantages inherent in hospitalization.

The treatment may sometimes consist of fatherly advice and at other times a more or less deep psychotherapy. In the latter case, once again the child-guidance services are the most suitable for the task.

Outpatient treatment is specially suitable for the youngest delinquents, at the very first signs of their antisocial behaviour, for at this moment aggressiveness has not yet assumed its more violent forms, and can be treated and resolved without any disturbing behaviour occurring which the family and society cannot tolerate. Later on, this is not always possible. The early treatment of such cases, independent of any legal or administrative procedure, is the advantage offered by child-guidance clinics, readily and freely available to the public.

In the course of such treatment an early social prognosis would be very helpful in order to take preventive steps in good time and to follow up their success. Glueck & Glueck's work[44] will be awaited with great interest as it sets out criteria for a social prognosis from the age of 8 years onwards.

> Of course, outpatient treatment can also be of great help to older patients, particularly if neurotic, or in whom neurotic factors have a large share in the genesis of their criminal tendencies.

Outpatient treatment, as I have shown, can take many forms, from psychotherapy to straightforward social and re-educational measures; but to be completely successful the psychology of the emotions should not be overlooked. It need not always be carried out by specialists in psychotherapy, though always with their collaboration. It is difficult to see the value of organizations where young delinquents are invited once or twice a week to see a film or have an hour's basket-ball, in the belief that almost by magic this will improve their relations with a law-abiding society.

Outpatient treatment has the further advantage of flexibility. If necessary, other members of the delinquent's family can be taken on, a brother or sister, over whom there is jealousy, and, above all, the parents, some of whose harmful attitudes can be modified. A family re-adjustment " in vivo " can be attempted, a procedure too often neglected when the delinquent is under detention. Outpatient treatment can also be combined with placing the delinquent in another family, or in a small hostel on licence.

4.4 Residential Treatment

The social worker who, throughout his professional life, is constantly sending young people to re-educational institutions must end by considering this a commonplace measure. No blame can be attached to him. But it is sometimes well to remember that each time a person resorts to such measures he ought to feel conscience-stricken. To bring this home he should ask himself this question: " Which re-educational institution among those known to me and where I often send delinquents, would I select, with a quiet mind, for my own boy or girl, if one of them had been so unfortunate as to commit a crime ? "

Of course, such institutions are essential. They are not merely a necessary evil, as some hold, for a few obtain encouraging positive results. But along with these results, how many failures occur due to faulty technique, how much aggressivity is unleashed, how often are the feelings of loneliness strengthened ? How many juveniles are exposed to degrading influences with daily loss of self-respect, tempted by perversions, or in the less striking cases, simply suffering from that sort of mental anaemia which affects all inmates of institutions, the result of living in a vacuum on meagre emotional rations ?

This having been said, there is no further need for a detailed criticism of re-educational programmes, or plans for the ideal re-educational institution. Remembering the aim and scope of this report I shall restrict myself to certain observations which from a psychiatric standpoint seem particularly important.

(1) It is the quality of the director and staff of an institution which above all else determines the value of the work carried on within it. It would be impossible to list exactly the qualities which each member of the staff of an institution should possess. It often seems as if pyknic personalities are the most suited to direct a reform institution ; on the other hand,

there are many excellent re-educators who have the temperament generally associated with the leptosomatic type. Some directors have an advanced knowledge of psychology, while others rely on their more practical gifts for teaching. While it is desirable to have on the staff subordinates with technical training and, above all, with a good standard of education, it is also quite definitely valuable to have one or two more forthright and simple personalities, with whom certain pupils find contact easier and more direct than with the more cultured re-educators. But most important of all, only the emotionally stable should be employed. Particular care should be taken to eliminate any psychopaths and psychoneurotics, who are only too often attracted to the re-education of these antisocial youths by a sort of positive tropism which must be uncovered. The following personalities should likewise be eliminated: homosexuals, either overt, or with strong latent tendencies, the dissatisfied, the over-possessive, the more or less openly sadistic and masochistic; in short, all whose activity in a reform institution, on careful psychological examination, to adopt a saying of Odier, [86] seems to serve a biological function necessary to satisfy their own neurosis, rather than the desire to be of service to a social ideal.

To insist that all members of the senior staff of a reform institution should themselves have been psycho-analysed is an unrealizable demand. And yet I am more and more convinced of the immense benefit to the re-educator of the knowledge acquired from such analysis, of self and of others. His relations with pupils, colleagues, superiors, and subordinates would thereby be greatly improved and his collaboration with the psychiatrist and the psychologist would become infinitely easier. In the absence of such training, a good knowledge of depth psychology should be insisted on in the senior staff.

It is very desirable that there should be a number of women on the staffs of these institutions for boys and adolescent youths. Similarly, in re-educational institutions for young and adolescent girls the possibility of positive transference relationship to a man as father-figure should be offered them.

(2) A reform institution should be organized in such a way that its pupils are divided into small families or groups. The ideal arrangement is found in certain Swedish and American reform institutions where each group, sometimes consisting of not more than seven children, lives in a cottage under the supervision of a trained married couple. Meals are prepared there, and the life closely resembles normal family life. It is also an advantage not to mix certain age-groups, particularly children of school-age with those of post-school age. On the other hand, within a group of school-age children the different ages can be mixed advantageously. An important point, upon which Aichhorn used to insist, is to take great care only to place pupils with a re-educator for whom they have a certain,

natural affinity, and he for them. Without such an affinity, it seems impossible to re-educate really successfully. I have been present at the weighty and learned discussions of the staff at reform institutions on a particular case, when it was clear the discussion was useless, since not one of the speakers felt any real sympathy with the case. When this happens there should be no hesitation in changing the child's group, or even sending him to another institution. The lack of sympathy in re-education brings on a mental anaemia which quickly becomes fatal.

While the reform institutions for children of pre-pubertal age can often profitably be co-educational, the general opinion seems to be that, from puberty onwards, it is better to segregate the sexes. However, the reform institution Cedar Knoll at Hawthorne, near New York City, run by the Jewish Board of Guardians, takes pupils of both sexes up to the age of 18, and results seem excellent.

Many opportunities for re-education are afforded by the " children's villages " or " children's republics " of which there are well known prototypes in Italy and the USA, but there are pitfalls, and it would be a mistake to think that they are the only satisfactory plans for a re-educational community. Here, as elsewhere, it is the attitude of the re-educators in charge that counts.

(3) There is much that could be said on the architectural layout of the buildings of a reform institution. Perhaps the mind can give life to stone, and good re-educational work be achieved under adverse material circumstances, but the influence of surroundings can be of the greatest help. Some thought should be given to the aesthetic side of these buildings, and one is all too often shocked to note its absence both in the USA and Europe. On both sides of the Atlantic I have seen buildings which were often hideously ugly, appallingly so, and have been surprised to find the latest cooking and refrigerating installations. The responsible committees do not seem to realize that, important as it is to help the cook in her work, it is sometimes more urgent to help the re-educators in theirs. Indeed the latter might be the less expensive outlay. This is especially true of reform institutions for girls—though it applies also to those for boys. How can these girls be taught to be tidy, to look after a house, to like pleasant, well-kept living conditions, if they are constrained to live in such a sordid atmosphere? In this way a powerful re-educational force is wasted.

Need it be said that all systems of cages still found in the dormitories of some reform institutions should be entirely done away with, as indeed, all bars on windows, locked doors, patrol galleries, enclosure walls, watchtowers, and the like. All the good re-educational centres I visited had long since done away with these archaic devices, without any disastrous consequences, even where somewhat difficult cases were concerned. Naturally there are a few really violent juvenile delinquents who need to be locked up, but there is absolutely no reason to apply to the immense majority of inmates a regime which is helpful only with a few, and harmful to the rest. These violent cases should be housed in specially built houses or else sent, with no more ado, to adult penal institutions—a step which can be justified on practical grounds, and which is certainly more reasonable than to allow all the inmates to suffer for two or three vicious elements.

(4) Throughout my professional life and everywhere on my tour, I met with the problem of escapes and the antagonism it creates between the re-educator, who understands that some escapes are inevitable if one really wishes to re-educate, and the police, and sometimes the general public, who react to any escape with cries of " anarchy ". It cannot be too strongly emphasized that such reactions are unfortunate, and spring from a complete misunderstanding of the facts. A delinquent's escape from an institution is an inevitable risk if one seeks truly to re-educate, and the directors must feel themselves upheld in this regard by superior authority and by public opinion.

(5) No up-to-date reform institution can be organized without regular psychological and psychiatric collaboration. It is, however, foolish to conceal the difficulties this entails. There is a certain antagonism between the views of the psychiatrist and the re-educator which must be recognized and admitted. While the re-educator seeks to impress a chosen behaviour pattern on his pupil, the psychiatrist seeks to make him express his inner drives. If psychiatrists and psychologists cannot work side by side, acknowledging that the work of one is complementary to that of the other, clashes will occur which result in the disruption of the institution's routine. I have already enlarged on this theme elsewhere and can therefore only briefly refer to it here.[9, 14]

In brief, there are three possible forms of collaboration between a reform institution on the one hand and the psychiatrist and psychologist on the other.

(*a*) Psychiatrists and psychologists can limit themselves to making a diagnosis. The director may sometimes send them all the pupils, as they enter, or only those cases which seem particularly difficult. After examination of these pupils, a written or verbal report is made to the director.

(*b*) The psychiatrist and psychologist can place themselves at the disposal of the director and his staff for joint discussion on difficult cases; they can indicate how they see the problems and their solution; they can try to make the re-educators aware of their personal difficulties, and how these may hinder their work; in short, they can act as psychological advisers to the staff of an institution.

(*c*) The psychiatrist and the psychologist, instead of limiting themselves to examining the pupils, or to giving advice to the staff, can maintain a close contact with the pupils or at least with some of them, which in effect amounts to giving psychotherapy of varying regularity and intensity.

These three methods here outlined are all equally suitable according to the circumstances in which the reform institution and consulting psychiatrist are placed.

Diagnostic work alone can be very valuable when the psychiatrist and psychologist have little time and when, for personal or technical reasons, a closer collaboration is difficult. This diagnosis however must not be limited to measuring the IQs. This is a danger which some reform institutions do not escape, though they pride themselves on employing one or more psychologists. It is necessary, therefore, to emphasize that, when a psychologist's work in an institution is confined to measuring IQs with the addition of a few projection tests, mechanically applied, it is incomplete, and even a waste of time, an illusion, an excuse for laziness on the part of the directors of the institution who fondly believe that they are meeting present-day demands by employing a psychologist, while remaining unaware that his work is useless because it leaves the essential points untouched. The work of a psychologist in these institutions, even when only diagnostic, must penetrate the whole personality of the pupil, revealing the depths of his mental life, exploring his unconscious, uncovering his constitutional tendencies, and taking his heredity into account. This requires time and patience and the collaboration of the psychiatrist with the psychologist. Even then there must be some assurance that the staff will read the reports with understanding and acceptance of their implications, and will be able to draw practical and appropriate conclusions.

It is clear that in order to do this work in the way I have just described, the second method of collaboration outlined above must be followed. Psychiatrists and psychologists should maintain as close and personal a contact as possible with the staff, being present at case conferences, always ready to help the re-educators find a solution to their problems, and should seek to inculcate a psychological approach. This task implies that psychiatrists and psychologists are completely familiar with the re-educator's problems, that they have easy social contacts and are adaptable, and that they are both modest and persevering. A serious stumbling-block is the anxiety of many re-educators when first collaborating with a psychiatrist, an anxiety which easily changes into reactive aggression. Surprised by the complex processes revealed by the psychiatrist, disconcerted by knowledge of the delinquent's paradoxical reactions, the re-educator, overwhelmed by feelings of impotence and ignorance, will either give up, or take refuge more than ever in classical and superficial methods of schooling, whose simplicity reassures him. On the other hand, a re-educator's enthusiasm for psychological notions before he has properly digested them is also to be avoided: this is sometimes merely another form of resistance. Such a task is difficult, requiring the psychiatrist and psychologist to apply first to themselves and their own problems the knowledge they wish to communicate to others. With these reservations, I believe that this form of collaboration is extremely fruitful, and that it should become, in one form or another, the basic pattern for all collaboration between doctors, psychologists, and re-educators.

Some reform institutions have solved this problem by making a psychiatrist director. This can be an excellent solution, provided the psychiatrist has also a good re-educator at his side. It is not, however, essential except for schools which specialize in psychopathological cases.

Psychiatric and psychological collaboration, when it takes the form of psychotherapy of the pupils in an institution, presents great practical difficulties. Aichhorn himself, who certainly could not be accused of being against psychotherapy, often pointed out its drawbacks. These result from the problems of transference which are especially difficult since the psychotherapist is always considered more or less a member of the staff by the pupil. Moreover, psychotherapy sometimes lets loose temporary aggressive reactions and other antisocial manifestations, and creates disciplinary problems for the staff. It is therefore difficult to carry out such therapy if the staff are not very much alive to psychological problems, and have not themselves undergone an analysis if possible. Experience repeatedly shows, in any case, that conflicts are very frequent between the staff and the psychotherapist, the patient and the staff, and the patient and his companions.

In cases where such therapy is technically possible, the results are sometimes excellent. It will be especially interesting to follow the experiment, now in progress, at the Duncroft Reform Institution for girls, at Staines, near London, under the National Association for Mental Health; a parallel experiment with boys is about to be, or has already been, started. But I must add, in passing, that at the time of my visit to Duncroft, there were 8 staff for 11 inmates! Two psychiatrists carried out treatment on this small group. Only carefully selected psychoneurotics are accepted (constitutional psychopaths being excluded) with a minimum IQ of 80. From this may be seen the price the directors of this experiment are prepared to pay in order that the inmates should have the benefit of psychotherapy.

(6) The question of length of residential treatment is much under discussion today all over the world. Generally speaking, the re-educators insist on having their pupils for a considerable time, while magistrates, social workers, and psychiatrists show a tendency to shorten the length of stay. This tendency is gaining ground nowadays, and I have even heard a fair number of directors of institutions say also that the pupils' stay should be as short as possible. This is particularly felt to apply to the older pupils of post-school age, for whom a stay of 12 months is considered by many establishments as maximum, with 8-10 months as the optimum; while for children of school-age, two or three years is

considered suitable. It is difficult to make hard and fast rules, and these figures are only to give a general idea. It seems to me, though, that in the past we have sometimes thought that residential treatment has almost magical virtues, directly proportional to its duration. Each case must be judged individually, and it must be remembered that the institutional atmosphere, even the best, is artificial and there is great risk of mental anaemia. With good after-care available, and a few hostels for delinquents on licence (see page 74), the stay in institutions can often be shortened. I also consider that it is a mistake to think that a delinquent after a time at a reform institution, who on release commits a further crime, must necessarily begin his re-education all over again, and that he must be detained anew for a long time. Such relapses are sometimes the last signs of a resolving crisis, and do not always entail a further lengthy period of detention. If such a measure is thought desirable, two or three months may prove sufficient.

Great care must be taken with the many adolescents who, before committing some crime, have already lived for years in homes for lost children, orphanages, etc. There are frequently to be found in these reform institutions boys and girls of 16, 17, or 18, who have been for many years in institutions, sometimes even since birth, though perhaps under detention for only a short time. The re-educator's task here is to try once and for all to put such a stunted personality back into the stimulating everyday world even at the risk of some unfortunate lapses.

Since the idea of re-education has replaced that of punishment, it would seem logical to do away with the fixing of a set length of time for re-educative measures, and to make their duration depend on the delinquent's behaviour. But the psychology of the emotions knows not logic. In reality an indeterminate length for re-education and especially for residential treatment is a continual source of concern, anxiety, and resentment for the inmate of an institution. In many cases his uncertainty ruins his relations with the staff and authorities, and seriously hinders his real re-education. This is one of the points which the doctor must never tire of emphasizing to a magistrate, who, starting from a different point of view, believes on the contrary that only a stay of indefinite length will serve the purpose. It should not be impossible to find a compromise, satisfying both the reasonable demands of the law and the imperious needs of the emotions.

(7) The question of the relations between a reform institution and the parents is beginning to occupy the minds of many directors. This is as it should be. Some directors devote a considerable part of their time to interviewing the parents, often having a special office in some convenient place in the town, more accessible than the institution itself. Such contacts often help the re-educator to a better understanding of his pupils. Furthermore, these interviews have a good effect on the parents and may help the child by clarifying his situation in regard to his family. Experience shows that it is often useful to have such contacts even with so-called " bad " parents, and that this is the best means of helping the child to become at last independent of them, since his ambivalent feelings of love and hate towards them prevent his social adjustment.

(8) Release from the reform institution must be much better prepared for than it is generally. Too often after several months, if not years, in an institution, the delinquent's behaviour is finally satisfactory, and he is then thrown without preparation into the difficulties and temptations of the outside world. All the less prepared because of his life in the artificial institution atmosphere, frequently having stored up a good measure of aggression against society during his detention, highly vulnerable in his self-esteem, and disliking the slightest mention of his past, the adolescent thus put back into circulation is very likely to relapse, or worse, he will adopt a way of life which, while remaining on the right side of the law, will nevertheless leave him chronically maladjusted. The transition from the regime of the reform institution to the regime of life in the normal world should therefore be carefully prepared. To this end it is worth while to give the pupil several leaves before his final release. While still under detention the delinquent should be put in touch with a future employer or with the social agency who will take care of him when he comes out, so that, once he is free, he will not have to deal with strange people only. Some reform institutions have special sections where the adolescents before leaving have a thorough training in independence and responsibility. Whatever methods are chosen, the important point is that the institution's staff should recognize this as a problem, which, if not taken into account, can result in the waste of painstaking efforts.

4.5 Delinquents on Licence

The prominent feature of the system of putting juvenile delinquents on licence is that he is not restricted in his activities for twenty-four hours out of twenty-four, but can lead a part of his daily life as freely as other young people of his own age and class.

The common practice is that the delinquent on licence spends his nights and leisure hours in an institution, with a flexible discipline, while working in a school, workshop, or office like any other pupil, apprentice, or employee, leading a normal life. The system could also work the other way round: the delinquent, living at home and spending his free time there, but working in a school or workshop, specially planned for the re-education of the maladjusted. This "reversed licence system" is practised for example, by the public institution called Basler Webstube, in Basle (Switzerland) and has proved itself of great value with cases where the delinquent was well adjusted to his family, but maladjusted to his profession or job.

The licence system most often used (where the juvenile lives in an institution, but works outside) can take three different forms:

(1) A reform institution can place some of its pupils on licence, without any change in its internal organization, the licensed delinquents mixing with the pupils who have not this advantage.

(2) A reform institution may have a special division, more or less apart from the main building, where licensed delinquents are transferred.

(3) Special institutions may be organized solely for delinquents on licence : the English and American hostel system.

The first form has serious disadvantages. Many directors are hostile to it, while others treat it as a makeshift. There are, however, a number of reform institutions, particularly in the USA, Sweden, and Switzerland, where this system is in force, to the satisfaction of all. Generally speaking, however, either separate hostels, or a department for delinquents on licence within an institution, with its own separate life, are preferable.

The advantages of the system of putting delinquents on licence stand out particularly in the following examples :

(1) When a juvenile delinquent has already begun an apprenticeship, and when none of the reform institutions to which he could be sent has the necessary workshop where his particular speciality can be learnt, this system will save him from breaking off his apprenticeship.

(2) This system can be used as a transition from living in a closed institution to complete freedom, and is part of the after-care measures to be described later.

(3) In the many cases where the home will not help the delinquent's complete social recovery on his discharge from the reform institution, hostels provide an excellent solution more easily acceptable to the family and to the delinquent himself than the provision of a foster-home in the same town.

(4) A department for delinquents on licence, within a reform institution, can often become a useful holiday centre or place of refuge for ex-pupils. Some people derive considerable help from the knowledge that they can spend a few days at any time in an understanding atmosphere.

(5) Finally, hostels situated in the centre of big towns can be used as restaurants or clubs by the inmates of country reform institutions who come into the town to work.

The use of a hostel or special division for delinquents on licence must conform to a number of technical rules, which cannot be discussed in detail here. It is sufficient to say that the number of delinquents should not exceed 15 to 20 and that they should preferably be under the aegis of a married couple.

4.6 After-Care

As I have already said, after residential treatment, however apparently successful, a delinquent may quickly relapse if he is not suitably helped on his release. Ways of preparing his release have already been indicated. It is necessary to stress anew that it is of the greatest importance to follow the convalescent steps of the newly liberated delinquent for a time.

The consultative commission on juvenile delinquency of the International Union for Child Welfare spent part of its time on the study of this problem when it met at Beaumont-sur-Oise in April 1950.[64] I cannot do better than to quote some of its conclusions :

" After-care must consist of positive action to help the individual understand his problems, accept his responsibilities, and find a solution to his difficulties. It must not be merely an occasional and authoritarian supervision, or a rigid and routine system of control.

"After-care is an integral part of rehabilitation; there must be no hiatus in the continuity between residential treatment and the subsequent re-education for life in the outside world.

"Some countries have been successful in entrusting the supervision of discharged juvenile delinquents to the personnel of the institutions which they have left, provided the personnel has the necessary time.

"If not, or in addition, specially trained social workers should be used. They should be well paid, and should look after only a limited number of cases (maximum 50).

"These workers should have a knowledge of institutional life and should be in contact with the director of the institution and the members of the staff who were in charge of the delinquent. Voluntary workers can be very useful, provided they are guided and directed by trained workers.

"In any case the delinquent must willingly accept the person placed in charge of him; better still, he should have a certain freedom of choice, since confidence is essential between them. The delinquent must be allowed to take responsibility, to experiment for himself, even at the risk of slight relapses."

4.7 Training of Staff

Technical knowledge is indispensable for all who wish to work with juvenile delinquents, whether in recognizing them, in diagnosis, in prophylactic work, in outpatient or institutional treatment, or in supervision during after-care. Even more essential are a good level of general education, and emotional stability. All this implies that the selection and training of staff are of the greatest importance. Only hesitant beginnings have been made in this respect. Only in England and the USA are there a few efficient training schools for psychiatric social workers, which have gained a reputation for providing a really practical and useful training. In other directions, unfortunately, no such progress has been made.

The training of child psychiatrists is too often left to chance, or to attempts at self-instruction. There are excellent centres for the training of child psychotherapists but which cannot train enough highly qualified candidates. The position is better for the training of diagnostic psychologists. But this is not perhaps a speciality which plays any great part in juvenile delinquency. The most difficult problem is undoubtedly the training of staff of reform institutions. Remarkable experiments, such as the training centre at Amersfoort, in the Netherlands, are unfortunately few and far between. While a few institutions have a qualified staff, the vast majority, in Europe and the USA, have a personnel certainly not lacking in good-will, but whose mental stability and technical knowledge leave much to be desired.

The consultative commission on the delinquent and maladjusted child of the International Union for Child Welfare spent some time at its Amersfoort meeting in 1949 on this problem. Some of the resolutions adopted at this meeting seem to me to merit the attention of all those interested in this question. The foundation of training institutes for re-educators, the fixing of standards for awarding diplomas and the drawing-up of a charter for the staff, were all proposed as likely to ensure the necessary stability to a profession whose uncertain conditions had, till now, discouraged the most suitable candidates. It would take too long to quote all the resolutions here and I must refer the reader to the published proceedings of the Amersfoort [63] meeting which contain much important information.

4.8 Conclusions

If reference is made to the chapter on the etiology of juvenile delinquency, it will be clear that with such varied processes involved in the causation of juvenile delinquency, methods of re-education and treatment will also have to be very varied.

For example, cases where the super-ego is insufficiently developed have a very different structure from those where self-punishment mechanisms come into play, and where the super-ego seems, on the contrary, too unyielding and severe. Cases of slight retardation in mental development almost automatically improve, simply by means of the regular and ordered life in an institution, while the profound maladjustment of some passive personalities will remain untouched by this same procedure.

It is precisely because of this diversity of causes, requiring, in return, a diversity of measures, that psychiatric and psychological collaboration is indispensable at all stages and in all forms of treatment for juvenile delinquents. It is also the reason why it must be insisted that the unqualified staff, in whatever capacity they deal with juvenile delinquents, should have a minimum knowledge of psychology.

While, of course, other factors—social, family, legal—should be taken into account, the psychological structure of each case must be the basis for deciding on any particular measures: residential treatment or the placing of juvenile delinquents on licence; straightforward advice or psychotherapy; re-educational measures or medical treatment; superficial social measures or attempts at a fundamental change in the delinquent. Within the limits imposed by any of these measures each case must be individually dealt with. Psychotherapy, for example, cannot follow a rigid plan; it may be deep, more typical of adult psychotherapy, or rather more superficial, or make use of normal teaching methods. In the same way a rigid regime in reform institutions should be avoided and more pliable methods employed. This flexibility can be made much easier by organizing the institution in small groups or families, with diverse types of re-educators in charge, who differ from one another in temperament, interests, age, and sex. In their turn, the authorities responsible for the decisions taken about a delinquent should not hesitate in some cases to change a sentence of institutional detention to a placing of the delinquent on licence, or to remove a delinquent from a foster-home to institutional detention, or to substitute individual treatment for general rehabilitation or vice versa, until by experimenting the right solution has been found.[1] Nevertheless, all the measures, advice, detention, psychotherapy, or any other procedure applied to a delinquent have a common aim; this primary aim is to foster the growth in the delinquent of stable, secure, emotional relations with some person who gains his confidence. By whatever paths, in fact, the delinquent arrives at delinquency, we find in the factors leading to crime a common denominator in the following vicious circle: insecurity, anxiety, aggression, guilt, insecurity. In the same way, the common denominator of therapy is security rediscovered. It is in living through the experience of a sound relationship with the re-educator or therapist, based on mutual respect, and preserving the individuality of both, that the juvenile will find this security anew.[m]

In a pamphlet edited by the Jewish Board of Guardians [66] of New York, I found the following passage which seems to me to illustrate very clearly the importance of this process:

" Part of the treatment of many children consists of helping them to develop genuine affection for the worker [or for the re-educator, therapist, etc.]. To love is to be vulnerable, whether it is between child and parents, between man and woman, between friends—or client and therapist. Poets have described it, scientists have proved it and everybody knows it. It is to place one's vital happiness at the mercy of another, to expose the most sensitive feelings to the possibility of abiding pain should this reaching out to another person be met with coolness or outright rebuff. Yet, without the capacity for affection, no permanent or deep happiness or contentment is possible." Maladjusted children " have had over and over again in their own lives the painful experience of being disappointed and frustrated in their close attachments, usually in their immediate family, and they fear to repeat this experience. Since such a child suffers from an inability to enter warm and satisfying relationships with other people, it becomes the task of the case worker to give him the experience of exchanging trust and affection with another person. The child is truly helped when he can permit himself to feel and to display affection once more and to find out that, although hurt may be in the offing, there is also potential happiness and growth in relinquishing the inward bitterness which had prevented a wholesome, energetic approach toward life; in its stead is substituted a readiness to like other people, a warmth and richness of feeling which are the essentials for a creative and happy life."

The basic aim of all treatment could not be better epitomized.

---

[1] The Swiss penal code, in Articles 86 and 93, takes this into account in stating " the competent authority can, at any time, substitute another measure for the one ordered ".

[m] The work of the brilliant Russian educator, Makavenko, [49, 50] whose opinions otherwise diverge from those given here, shows in this respect ideas similar to those held in the best Western institutions.

SUMMARY AND GENERAL CONCLUSIONS

To conclude this report, I shall try to summarize the main points and draw a number of conclusions. I shall therefore review each chapter, recapitulating the essential outlines, emphasizing the basic and proved facts, and, finally, indicating the principal fields in which further research appears necessary.

1.1 Juvenile delinquency is an artificial concept, legal and social in origin. Psychologically, it involves social "disadaptation" or maladjustment. But all socially maladjusted people are not delinquents, and all delinquents are not socially maladjusted.

Nevertheless, to be brought before a juvenile court and to be subjected to various measures creates a number of psychological reactions which delinquents have in common and which give a secondary psychological homogeneity to an otherwise heterogeneous group.

The artificial nature of the concept of delinquency varies, in particular, according to the laws in force or to the way in which they are applied, and this makes it extremely difficult to establish statistical comparisons between one country and another, or one period and another. This is a major obstacle to research and a possible source of serious error.

Since there is no question of unifying the laws of all countries, it is desirable that statistics on juvenile delinquency should have uniform criteria and should give a clear and detailed picture of the various kinds of offences to which they relate. The establishment of such norms is an urgent task.

1.2 One of the most definite conclusions of this investigation is that few fields exist in which more serious coercive measures are applied, on such flimsy objective evidence, than in that of juvenile delinquency.

This paucity of evidence is due to material and psychological factors. The psychological factors can be eliminated by a personal effort, on the part of all research workers in juvenile delinquency, to become increasingly objective; material difficulties could be overcome if public authorities and other interested groups would make available the funds necessary for research.

In view of the enormous financial burden which delinquency imposes on a population (about 100 million Swiss francs annually for a country such as Switzerland), it would seem reasonable to devote annually a sum for research, if only as a kind of insurance premium.

2.1 For more than half-a-century two etiological concepts—the organic and the psychogenic—have been in continuous opposition. It is absolutely essential that this should cease and that research be orientated to the study of the ways in which constitution and environment, soma and psyche, are always involved in the manifestations of social maladjustment. When constitutional reasons are advanced as an explanation of some particular behaviour, it should be remembered that an individual's biological soil contains not only an hereditary contribution, but also the concretions of all the physical and psychological influences experienced throughout life.

The developmental studies, such as those of Freud and Piaget in particular, explain why it is relatively much easier for a juvenile than for an adult to cross, sometimes even without noticing, the comparatively low threshold which separates social maladjustment from delinquency. Not until the ultimate stages of the individual's psychological and moral development are completed—which may not be until after adolescence—does this threshold reach its final level.

2.2 Everyday observation, confirmed by numerous studies from the USA, Great Britain, and Germany after the first World War, points to the etiological importance of the environment, without the intermediary action of complex psychological mechanisms. A large proportion of children and adolescents appearing before the courts have no major physical or psychological abnormality. They are simply the victims of adverse external circumstances, characterized by social insecurity or a too low standard of living, or a combination of both. But for such social factors to cause delinquency, they must set in motion a number of psychological processes.

At present so little is known about these problems that it would be of the greatest practical interest to learn more, since social action is sometimes easier than psychological action. Hence experiments such as those carried out by the Chicago Area Project in the USA and the Institute for the Scientific Treatment of Delinquency in England deserve encouragement and should be copied elsewhere.

2.3 Numerous misunderstandings and a certain confusion exist today concerning the concept of constitutional psychopathy and its relation to antisocial behaviour. It is well to realize that this term does not have the same meaning in all countries, and that its sense changes from one side of the Atlantic to the other.

It is therefore urgent that there should be an agreed definition of the terms in use.

Modern research on the physiology of the autonomic nervous system, the growing knowledge of the electro-encephalograph, and recent advances in the incompatibility of blood factors, of foetal infections, and of anatomical or physiological traumata at birth, all help to complete ideas of the part played by somatic factors in the genesis of antisocial behaviour.

Genetic research, the comparison of twins in particular, should give most interesting results, especially when conducted on a large scale, which, however, requires considerable financial resources.

The correlation between mental deficiency and delinquency, which was accepted for a long time without question, is today much debated.

Here also, new studies, taking into account all possible sources of error, should be undertaken. In such studies particular attention should be paid to the fact that the juvenile delinquents confined to institutions, and even all those brought before a court, are only a fraction, sometimes rather artificially selected, of all socially maladjusted juveniles.

Already it seems likely that, other things being equal, the mental defective more easily becomes a victim of unfavourable social and psychological circumstances, owing to his mental instability and suggestibility. It is certain that if mental deficiency is found together with a psychopathic constitution, the prognosis is extremely poor. Finally, experience shows that it is absolutely essential to place mentally defective delinquents together in special institutions.

The etiological importance of organic disease and disabilities is very variable. Syphilis is no longer considered as important as formerly. Head injuries in children before puberty have a good prognosis. Certain forms of encephalitis, though sometimes subclinical, may contribute to an antisocial-behaviour syndrome assumed to be constitutional. Whilst epilepsy itself plays in practice only a minor role in the etiology of delinquency, the epileptic temperament is considered by some European writers to be not unimportant in the genesis of crime.

In general, organic disease is not of overwhelming importance in the etiology of antisocial behaviour. It would be inexpedient to limit the activities of the psychiatrist to the examination and treatment of these cases only.

2.4 Disturbances in the psychological development of personality which can play a part in the etiology of juvenile delinquency can be summarized briefly as follows:

2.4.1 Qualitative defects of the super-ego: For various reasons the superego of the child, though formed in accordance with the normal rules of personality development, may contain an antisocial element which may lead the child into delinquent behaviour.

2.4.2 Partial retardation of development: The formation of the ego may be delayed. In this respect, developmental disorders springing from some disturbance of normal mother and baby relationships are particularly important. Research into the consequences, at a later age, of early emotional frustration seems specially useful and needs further development. Some work, particularly in Great Britain and the USA, has already been done, and WHO is at this moment sponsoring an important investigation on this subject.

The formation of the super-ego, like that of the ego, may also be retarded or hindered by partial retardation of development.

2.4.3 Psychoneurosis and isolated psychoneurotic symptoms: While the fully fledged psychoneuroses do not, in practice, appear to play a very important part in the genesis of juvenile delinquency, this is certainly not the case with a number of isolated, neurotic symptoms: compulsions, need for self-punishment, symbolic expression of repressed urges, primary or reactive aggression, feeling of being abandoned and its various consequences —all such factors and many others play a considerable part in the genesis of much antisocial juvenile behaviour. It is essential for all who deal with juvenile delinquents to have a thorough, basic knowledge of this subject; without such knowledge, many delinquent cases will remain incomprehensible and the measures adopted will be totally inadequate.

2.4.4 Psychoses and "the psychotic reaction pattern": Before puberty, true psychosis is rare and plays almost no part in the etiology of delinquency. In the USA one sometimes finds a considerable role assigned to infantile and juvenile schizophrenia owing it seems to a wider use of the term than is customary in Europe. Without prejudging the issue, perhaps it could be said that psychological disorders can conform to a " psychotic reaction pattern " typified by the breakdown of relations between the instincts, the ego, and the super-ego, when the instinctual impulses, imperfectly controlled or repressed, break into the ego, and the adaptation to reality is thereby seriously disturbed.

2.5 The influence of the cinema, radio, and press is very often considered pernicious. An objective study of the facts has led to the conclusion that this is a more or less likely hypothesis, as yet unverified.

The cinema, radio, and press are certainly very important influences which force themselves on the attention of the public, and of young people particularly, by their special advertising methods. Completely objective research is still required to estimate their influence exactly, and also to see how far they could be used for educational purposes. Some such research is in progress in Europe and the USA but it needs to be intensified and made more systematic.

The same applies to the influence of leisure, about which little is known and which is the subject of a special research project by the Institute for the Scientific Treatment of Delinquency.

The disastrous consequences of alcoholism result chiefly from the psychological effects of alcoholic parents on the home atmosphere. It represents a real scourge, particularly in some European countries. On the other hand, it is necessary to be critical in assigning any importance to the so-called alcoholic heredity, which recent genetic studies suggest to be dubious.

2.6 The diversity of the etiological factors which have been enumerated leads to the classification of juvenile delinquency as a bio-psycho-social phenomenon (Lafon). It must be studied and attacked from these three angles. The psychiatrist, whose training is both biological and psychological, with his interest in social problems, and with the knowledge he should have of interhuman relationships, could play a useful part in co-ordinating the efforts of the different specialists in juvenile delinquency and in helping them to work together with mutual understanding.

Since this report sets out to examine the psychiatric aspects of juvenile delinquency, the question arises as to whether this approach to the problem enables any general principle or common denominator of delinquency's threefold origin—biological, psychological, and social—to be distinguished. It seems to the author that this psychological common denominator can be found in the feeling of insecurity to which any criminal tendency, from whatever source, gives rise. Insecurity gives rise, in its turn, to anxiety. Anxiety, by well-known psychological processes, tends to set free aggressiveness. This aggressiveness can take various forms; although sometimes very slight, it may also express itself by delinquent acts of all kinds, from the most harmless to the most serious. In most people, this aggressiveness will give rise to feelings of guilt which, in turn, produce further anxiety. Thus the vicious circle is completed which is doubtless one of the most constantly found psychological aspects of delinquency, particularly of juvenile delinquency.

3.1 It is generally admitted that the object of preventing juvenile delinquency is to lower the rate of adult delinquency. But the statistics show that only 10% to 20% of juvenile delinquents appearing before a court are future adult delinquents. Should prophylactic measures therefore be limited to this small minority?

If so, it would be necessary, in the first place, to be in a position to forecast which of the delinquents on trial are destined to become recidivists. A series of studies has been undertaken for the solution of this problem, and two important books, one by Glueck & Glueck,[44] in the USA, and the other by Frey, in Switzerland, both following previously published papers by these authors, will give the results of a long series of studies on this subject. In addition, the national inquiry on juvenile delinquency under the direction of Doctors G. Heuyer and L. Le Guillant now in progress in Paris is a research project of considerable importance which will also help to throw light on this problem.[108] Many more research projects, with control groups, are still needed.

But even if it proves possible to pick out those delinquents who are likely to become recidivists, this does not solve all the problems relating to prevention. To what extent are these cases accessible to preventive measures? If it proves possible to prevent them from committing crimes when young, will this stop them from committing them at a later age? Of these problems little is known, and prevention, when conceived only from the standpoint of preventing adult crime, raises a host of questions still to be answered.

Prevention can, however, be viewed from another angle. Just as the fight against tuberculosis has grown into a veritable public-health crusade, so the prevention of juvenile delinquency offers a unique opportunity to rally organizations and individuals with very diverse views under a common flag for a mental health crusade. If all the possible sources of juvenile delinquency are considered, it is clear that its prevention covers the whole field of mental health. For this reason the cantonal authorities of Vaud (Switzerland) have attached to the Département de Justice et Police a child-guidance unit, which deals with the whole range of child psychiatry and tries to spread appropriate child-guidance doctrines, only a small part of its total activities being devoted to real juvenile delinquents.

3.2 The sociological aspects of prevention concern the psychiatrist only in so far as he can indicate to the sociologist those aspects of the latter's work which seem to be of most psychological importance. In this connexion it seems that priority should be given to all those measures which enable a mother to be constantly with her child from birth and during the first three years at least. Much recent work with an immediate bearing on this subject has been directed to the study of the severe, and often irreversible, consequences with regard to later social adaptation that follow emotional deprivation in the first few years of a child's life.

Problems of housing, holidays, and communities fostering delinquency are also very important.

3.3 The prevention of constitutional psychopathy, in its narrow sense, can be based only on eugenic measures. The lack of theoretical knowledge, and a variety of moral and social reasons today prevent the application of such measures on a large scale.

In practice, the problem is not so much to prevent a psychopathic predisposition itself as to prevent its manifestations in a given individual under a given set of circumstances. Here the use of social psychiatry, through child-guidance or through public mental health services, would be of great help.

Although little is known of the correlation between mental deficiency and delinquency, experience seems to show that through special teaching the social adjustment of mental defectives can be immensely improved. The number of special classes for these cases needs to be increased and institutions to which they may be sent when they cannot be brought up by their own families improved.

Organic disease and disabilities may favour social maladjustment owing to "hospitalism", which often follows prolonged stay in hospitals or sanatoria. The all too permissive and yet frustrating atmosphere of these institutions can seriously affect the growth of a child's character. Similarly, though slightly different psychological processes are involved, disastrous consequences may follow prolonged hospitalization of very young children. In either case, the closest co-operation between paediatrician or general practitioner on the one hand, and psychiatrist on the other, appears necessary.

3.4 Prevention of disturbances in the psychological development of the personality is a true psychiatric task. Here, the whole range of techniques will be used, from benevolent advice on psychological lines to real psychotherapy. Special attention should be given to the psychology of the parents and to all family factors. It is well to remember, however, that simple advice given to parents is rarely sufficient. Child-guidance workers, psychologists, and psychiatrists must reach the deeper emotional levels of the parents' personal problems to effect, by one method or another, the necessary readjustments. As an example of this, advice to young mothers, such as that given in England, is especially valuable. Mention must also be made of other social experiments such as that of the Rochester Child Health Institute (USA) which, with the object of prophylaxis and research, seeks to follow up every child in the population as completely as possible, taking into account both the physical and psychological aspects of the child's personality, together with his home and school difficulties.

While it seems reasonable that primary efforts should be directed to infancy and early childhood, school age and adolescence should naturally not be neglected.

3.5 As yet too little is known of the effects of the cinema, radio, and press to formulate preventive measures. Since, however, these commercialized sensory and emotional mental stimuli forcibly impose themselves on the public's mental life, and particularly on the adolescent's, it is very desirable that, in return, re-educators and psychiatrists should investigate the effects of these new forces and should decide on the steps necessary to render them innocuous, or even to enlist their aid in the building-up of the personality. These investigations should lead, sooner or later, to legislation, particularly on the minimum age of admission to some films, and on the criteria of film censorship.

Prevention in connexion with alcoholism is a vast and urgent task.

3.6 The major preventive tasks outlined above can be brought to a successful conclusion only by doctors, psychologists, social workers, re-educators, and magistrates working together in teams. Only in a " multidimensional " view of juvenile delinquency, with corresponding " multidimensional " prophylaxis, can there be any hope of overcoming all these difficult problems. One of the most effective ways of obtaining this co-operation is through child-guidance teams such as exist today in some parts of Europe and the USA.

4.1 It must always be remembered that measures applied to delinquents do not work by magic; their success depends on us. If it can be ensured that these measures do no harm, at least something useful will have been achieved. The separation of a juvenile from his family is a very serious step, which, though often useful and sometimes inescapable, can cause harm, and should therefore only be taken with the greatest caution.

It is surprising to discover how few good studies exist which try to ascertain psychological influence on juvenile delinquents of their stay in re-educational centres and the like. Further research is urgently needed on this point.[n]

4.2 The multiplicity of factors causing delinquency and the consequent diversity of therapeutic methods in use make observation and examination of each juvenile delinquent an absolute necessity.

In many cases this may be brief and may be included in the course of the usual investigations. It may be left to the magistrate responsible for the case, and hence the child can remain in the care of his family.

However, when there is the slightest doubt either about the reasons for a delinquent's behaviour, or about the suitability, or otherwise, of a particular measure, the necessity for a full clinical and psychological examination is paramount.

Such a clinical examination can often be held in an outpatient department and the harmful effects of detention thus avoided. There will be times when it proves impossible not to detain a juvenile, but this action should not be resorted to without previous psychiatric examination as an outpatient.

As a general rule, residential observation must take place in centres specially designed for this purpose.

The question of the techniques to be used in such observation centres raises a number of psychological problems, particularly since it is almost impossible to keep observation and re-education apart.

The perfecting of these techniques is an important task, and the correct solution to the problem lies in teamwork among magistrates, re-educators, and psychiatrists.

4.3 Provided the necessary technical resources are available, outpatient treatment of juvenile delinquents will often meet with success, thereby making for financial economies and avoiding the disadvantages inherent in hospitalization.

This outpatient treatment can advantageously be entrusted to child-guidance teams including doctors, psychologists, and social workers.

4.4 Institutional treatment should be used only after careful thought and for very definite reasons; for, while such treatment is often necessary and gives good results, it is not always successful and may lead to outbursts of aggressiveness and reinforce the delinquent's feeling of being forsaken.

The most important factor in any re-educational institution is the quality of the director and his staff. Too much care cannot be taken in the selection and training of such staff; and consequently, by implication, the personnel should have a status worthy of its functions.

The reform school should be so run as to allow its pupils to be divided into small groups or families. In so doing care must be taken to assign to a teacher only pupils with whom there is some reciprocal affinity.

---

[n] The national French inquiry on maladjusted children, now being made under the direction of Dr. G. Heuyer and Dr. L. Le Guillant, is an extensive work. Its results should be of great interest in relation to these questions. [108]

In general, too little attention is paid to the interior decoration of reform institutions; this is an important factor, especially in institutions for girls.

It seems to be irrational to submit the majority of the inmates in a reform institution to a strict regime which, though suitable for a few, is clearly harmful in its effects on the rest. If special, small houses are provided for the really violent cases, then for the others the family atmosphere can be created which is still too often today lacking in many schools, but which is, however, a powerful re-educational force.

If the aim of a reform institution is to develop, through the use of rational educational methods, a delinquent's sense of responsibility, then a certain number of escapes is quite inevitable; and all who have administrative and police responsibilities must understand that this is a fundamental risk in re-educational work. To try to prevent escapes must lead to bad re-education.

It is impossible to conceive a modern reform institution without the active co-operation of psychiatrists and psychologists. This co-operation can be obtained in a variety of ways. If, however, it is limited to the formality of routine intelligence-testing by a psychologist or psychiatrist, it will lose most of its value, and a false impression will be created that the psychological requirements of the situation are being met. Any psychological investigation which does not include the psychology of the emotions is inadequate.

Psychotherapy, as such, is difficult in institutions, though various experiments are now in progress which should be watched with interest.

In general, collaboration between re-educators and psychiatrists raises complex problems, requiring of both the exercise of great tact and mutual understanding in their solution.

On all sides the problem of the length of stay in an institution is under discussion. It seems to be generally agreed now that the optimum length of stay for delinquents of post-school age is 8 to 10 months, while for those of school-age it may be as long as 2 or 3 years.

There is a mistaken belief that if a delinquent, who has been for a time at a reform institution, commits a new offence after being released, his re-education must begin all over again and he must be further detained for a prolonged period. Such relapses are sometimes the last sign of a resolving crisis.

To detain a juvenile for an indefinite length of time often makes him feel insecure and anxious, with harmful effects. Magistrates and psychiatrists should between them find a solution to the problem of length of stay which is legally and psychologically satisfactory.

It is very important to develop and maintain a close contact between the reform institution and the parents.

The delinquent's release from the reform institution also needs careful preparation.

4.5 The practice of putting juvenile delinquents on parole can be used with advantage for those who wish to continue an apprenticeship—an impossibility whilst under detention. It can also be used as an intermediate stage between leaving an institution and being allowed full freedom. It may help when the home conditions of a discharged delinquent are unsuitable.

The use of a hostel for delinquents on parole should be determined by well-defined criteria; special qualities are required of its warden.

4.6 Juvenile delinquents from reform institutions, though apparently treated successfully, may quickly relapse if they are not guided after their discharge. Hence, after-care is an integral part of re-education and has to be systematically organized.

4.7 It is absolutely necessary for all who deal with juvenile delinquency, in whatever capacity, to acquire some technical knowledge, to have a good standard of general education, and to be emotionally stable.

The training of staffs for reform schools raises acute and difficult problems, and it is desirable that it should be undertaken in special schools. The personnel should have contracts guaranteeing stable financial conditions in return for the heavy burden of responsibility they have to bear.

4.8 Treatment should be adapted to each individual juvenile delinquent and should be based on the fundamental laws of psychology, particularly in its emotional and subconscious aspects.

In some cases there should be no hesitation in trying out a variety of methods until the one best suited to each individual's temperament and circumstances is found.

Even the most diverse methods have a common, primary aim—namely, that of enabling a juvenile delinquent to build up stable and secure interhuman emotional relations, the proof of a feeling of inner security which is itself a foundation for his moral independence and consideration for others, and without which no human behaviour can be truly adapted to the demands of society.

BIBLIOGRAPHY

Publications giving a general survey of the subject of this review and also those with extensive bibliographies are marked with an asterisk.

1. Ahnsjö, S. (1941) *Acta paediatr., Stockh.* **28**, Suppl. III
*2. Aichhorn, A. (1925) *Verwahrloste Jugend*, Wien
*3. Aichhorn, A. (1935) *Wayward youth*, New York (translation of 2)
4. Alexander, F. & Healy, W. (1935) *Roots of crime : psychoanalytic studies*, New York
5. Bender, L. (1947) *Psychopathic behavior disorders in children*. In : *Handbook of correctional psychology*, New York
6. Beno, N., Bersot, H. & Bovet, L. (1947) *Les enfants nerveux, leur dépistage et leur traitement par les services médico-pédagogiques*, Neuchâtel & Paris
7. Bergier, J. (1950) *Inform. Serv. Trav. soc.* **19**, 36
8. Bolterauer, L. (1947) *Rev. int. Enfant*, **11**, 113
9. Bovet, L. (1944) *Z. Kinderpsych.* **11**, 39
10. Bovet, L. (1947) *Schweiz. Aerzteztg.* **28**, 543
11. Bovet, L. (1948) *Schweiz. Aerzteztg.* **29**, 2
12. Bovet, L. (1948) In : *International Congress on Mental Health, London, 1948*, **2**, 88
13. Bovet, L. (1949) *Gesundh. Wohlf.* **29**, 285
14. Bovet, L. (1949) *Z. Kinderpsych.* **16**, 69
15. Bowlby, J. (1940) *Int. J. Psycho-Anal.* **21**, 154
*16. Bowlby, J. (1946) *Forty-four juvenile thieves, their characters and homelife*, London
17. Bowlby, J. (1951) *Bull. World Hlth Org.* **3**, 355
18. Brantmay, H. (1946) *Z. Kinderpsych.* **13**, 65
*19. Burt, C. (1948) *The young delinquent*, 4th ed. London
*20. Carr-Saunders, A. M., Mannheim, H. & Rhodes, E. C. (1942) *Young offenders, an enquiry into juvenile delinquency*, London
21. Chassell, C. (1935) *The relation between morality and intellect*, New York (Teachers Colleges Contribution to Education, No. 607, p. 133)
*22. Chazal, J. (1946) *Les enfants devant leurs juges*, Paris
23. Clinard M. B. (1949) *Ann. Amer. Acad. polit. soc. Sci.* **261**, 42
*24. Debesse, M. (1942) *L'adolescence*, Paris
25. Debesse, M. (1948) *Comment étudier les adolescents*, 3ᵉ éd. Paris
26. Debesse, M. (1948) *La crise d'originalité juvénile*, 3ᵉ éd. Paris
27. Debesse, M. *Hébélogie* (to be published)
*28. Eissler, K. R., ed. (1949) *Searchlights on delinquency. New psycho-analytic studies dedicated to Professor A. Aichhorn*, New York
29. Elliott, M. A. (1939) *Correctional education and the delinquent girl*, Philadelphia
*30. Exner, F. (1939) *Kriminalbiologie in ihren Grundzügen*, Hamburg
31. Freud, A. (1948) In : *International Congress on Mental Health, London, 1948*, **2**, 16
*32. Freud, A. (1949) *Le moi et les mécanismes de défense*, Paris
33. Frey, E. (1944) *Schweiz. Z. Strafrecht*, **58**, 277, 514
34. Frey, E. (1946) *Schweiz. Z. Strafrecht*, **60**, 70, 305
35. Frey, E. (1947) *L'avenir des mineurs délinquants*, Paris

36. Frey, E. (1949) *Biology and juvenile delinquency*, London (Howard League)
*37. Friedländer, K. (1947) *The psychoanalytical approach to juvenile delinquency*, London
38. Ganz, M. (1936) *La psychologie d'Alfred Adler et le développement de l'enfant*, Neuchâtel & Paris
39. Gemelli, A. (1948) *La personalità del delinquente nei suoi fondamenti biologici e psicologici*, ed. 2, Milano
40. Glueck, S. & Glueck, E. T. (1930) *500 criminal careers*, New York
41. Glueck, S. & Glueck, E. T. (1934) *Onè thousand juvenile delinquents*, Cambridge, Mass.
42. Glueck, S. & Glueck, E. T. (1936) *Preventing crime : a symposium*, New York
43. Glueck, S. & Glueck, E. T. (1940) *Juvenile delinquents grown up*, New York
44. Glueck, S. & Glueck, E. T. (1950) *Unraveling juvenile delinquency*, New York
45. Goddard, H. H. (1929) *J. juv. Res.* **13**, 262
46. Goldfarb, W. (1943) *J. exp. Educ.* **12**
47. Goldfarb, W. (1945) *Amer. J. Orthopsychiat.* **15**, 247
48. Goldfarb, W. (1945) *Amer. J. Psychiat.* **102**, 18
49. Goodman, W. L. (1949) *Anton Simeonovitch Makarenko, Russian teacher*, London
50. Grassberger, R. (1946) *Die Lösung kriminalpolitischer Probleme durch die mechanische Statistik*, Wien
51. Greef, E. de (1948) *Introduction à la criminologie*, Paris
52. Guex, G. (1949) *Rev. franç. Psychanal.* **13**, 257
53. Guex, G. (1950) *La névrose d'abandon*, Paris
*54. Guttmacher, M. S. (1949) *Bull. World Hlth Org.* **2**, 279
*55. Healy, W. & Bronner, A. F. (1936) *New light on delinquency and its treatment*, New Haven
56. Hess, W. R. (1924) *Schweiz. Arch. Neurol. Psychiat.* **15**
57. Hess, W. R. (1925) *Schweiz. Arch. Neurol. Psychiat.* **16**
58. Hess, W. R. (1948) *Die funktionelle Organisation des vegetativen Nervensystems*, Basel
59. Heuyer, G. (1946) *Rev. Educ. surv.* mai-juin
60. Hill, J. D. N. & Parr, G. (1950) *Electroencephalography. A symposium on its various aspects*, London
61. Hooton, E. A. (1939) *Crime and the man*, Cambridge, Mass.
62. International Congress of Psychiatry, Paris, 1950. Tome VI. Génétique et eugénique (reports by Kallmann, Penrose, Fraser Roberts, Slater, and Strömgren)
63. International Union for Child Welfare, Commission consultative de l'Enfance délinquante et socialement inadaptée (1949) *Rev. int. Enfant*, **13**, 93
64. International Union for Child Welfare, Compte rendu de la session de 1950 de la Commission consultative de l'Enfance délinquante et socialement inadaptée (to be published in *Rev. int. Enfant*)
65. International Union for Child Welfare, Conférence d'experts réunie à Genève et traitant des répercussions de la guerre sur la délinquance juvénile (1947) *Rev. int. Enfant*, **11**, 51
66. Jewish Board of Guardians (1948) *The story of the Jewish Board of Guardians*, New York
67. Joseph, B. (1948) *Brit. J. psychiat. soc. Work*, **2**, 30
*68. Joubrel, H. & Joubrel, F. (1946) *L'enfance dite coupable*, Paris
69. Kinberg, O. (1946) *Theoria*, **12**, 169
70. Kranz, H. (1936) *Lebensschicksale krimineller Zwillinge*, Berlin
*71. Lafon, R. (1950) *Psycho-pédagogie médico-sociale*, Paris

72. Lagache, D. (1946) *Rev. Educ. surv.* mai-juin
73. Lange, J. (1928) *Verbrechen als Schicksal*, Leipzig
74. Lebovici, S. (1949) *Rev. int. Filmol.* **2**, 49
75. Liévois, F. (1946) *La délinquance juvénile, cure et prophylaxie*, Paris
76. Lindner, R. M. (1945) *Rebel without a cause, the hypnoanalysis of a criminal psychopath*, London
77. Lutz, J. (1949) *Z. Kinderpsych.* **15**, 173 ; **16**, 97
78. Luxenburger, H. (1938) *Psychiatrische Erblehre*, München
79. McKay, H. D. (1949) *Ann. Amer. Acad. polit. soc. Sci.* **261**, 32
80. Makarenko, A. S. (1950) *Der Weg ins Leben, Ein pädagogisches Poem*, Berlin
*81. Mannheim, H. (1948) *Juvenile delinquency in an English middletown*, London
*82. Meng, H., ed. (1947) *Die Prophylaxe des Verbrechens*, Basel
83. Merrill, M. A. (1947) *Problems of child delinquency*, Boston
84. National Probation and Parole Association (1949) *A standard Juvenile Court Act*, rev. ed. New York
*85. *Nervous Child*, 1947, **6**, No. 4 (special number on juvenile delinquency)
86. Odier, C. (1947) *Les deux sources, consciente et inconsciente, de la vie morale*, 2ᵉ éd. Neuchâtel
87. Otterström, E. (1946) *Acta paediatr., Stockh.* **33**, Suppl. V
88. Parker, D. (1945) *Puissance et responsabilité du film*, Paris
89. Pearce, J. D. W. (1949) *The limits of present knowledge on juvenile delinquency*. In : *Why delinquency? ... Report of a conference on the scientific study of juvenile delinquency*, London
90. Piaget, J. (1926) *La représentation du monde chez l'enfant*, 1ᵉ éd. Paris
*91. Piaget, J. (1932) *Le jugement moral chez l'enfant*, 1ᵉ éd. Paris
92. Piaget, J. (1937) *La construction du réel chez l'enfant*, Neuchâtel & Paris
*93. Polier, J. W. (1941) *Everyone's children, nobody's child*, New York
94. Pollak, O. (1950) *J. crim. Law Criminol.* **40**, 701
95. Powers, E. (1949) *Ann. Amer. Acad. polit. soc. Sci.* **261**, 77
96. Probst, H. (1949) *Über psychische Folgen des Schädelbruches im Kindesalter* (Thesis, Zürich)
97. *Proceedings of the International Conference on Child Psychiatry, London, 1948*, London & New York, 1948 (*International Congress on Mental Health, London, 1948*, 2)
98. Ramer, T. (1946) *Acta psychiat., Kbh.* Suppl. 41
99. Reckless, W. C. (1943) *The etiology of delinquent and criminal behavior, a planning report for research*, New York (Social Science Research Council Bulletin, No. 50)
*100. Reckless, W. C. & Smith, M. (1932) *Juvenile delinquency*, New York
101. Reiwald, P. (1949) *Die Gesellschaft und ihre Verbrecher*, Zürich
102. Reiwald, P. (1949) *Society and its criminals*, London (translation of 101)
103. Repond, A. (1944) *Gesundh. Wohlf.* **24**, 193
*104. Repond, A. (1948) *Prophylaxie de la criminalité*, Bâle
105. Riggenbach, O. (1934) *Schweiz. Arch. Neurol. Psychiat.* **34**, 189
106. Rosanoff, A., Handy, L. M. & Rosanoff, I. (1941) *The etiology of child behavior difficulties, juvenile delinquency and adult criminality, with special reference to their occurrence in twins*, Sacramento, Calif. (California Department of Institutions, Psychiatric Monographs, No. 1)
107. Rubin, S. (1949) *Ann. Amer. Acad. polit. soc. Sci.* **261**, 1
108. *Sauvegarde de l'Enfance*, 1950, **5**, No. 3/4 (special number on juvenile delinquency)
109. Saxena, P. N. (1950) *Tribunal*, **1**, 10

110. Schneider, K. (1923) *Die psychopathischen Persönlichkeiten*, 1. Aufl. Wien; 8. Aufl. Wien, 1946
111. Sellin, T. (1938) *Culture conflict and crime*, New York (Social Science Research Council Bulletin, No. 41)
112. Shaw, C. R. (1930) *The jack-roller*, Chicago
113. Shaw, C. R. & McKay, H. D. (1931) *Social factors in juvenile delinquency*, Washington (National Commission on Law Observance and Enforcement, Report on causes of crime, 2, No. 13)
114. Shaw, C. R., McKay, H. D. & McDonald, J. F. (1938) *Brothers in crime*, Chicago
*115. Shaw, C. R., McKay, H. D. & McDonald, J. F. (1942) *Juvenile delinquency and urban areas*, Chicago
116. Sheldon, W. H. (1949) *Varieties of delinquent youth*, New York
117. Smith, M. (1947) *Rural Sociol.* September
*118. Solomon, B. (1947) *Juvenile delinquency, practical prevention*, Peekskill, N.Y.
119. Sorba, M. (1948) *Etudes de pathologie fœtale et néonatale*, Lausanne
120. Spitz, R. A. (1945) *Hospitalism : an inquiry into the genesis of psychiatric conditions in early childhood* [I]. In : *The psychoanalytic study of the child*, **1**, 53
121. Spitz, R. A. (1946) *Anaclitic depress on : an inquiry into the genesis of psychiatric conditions in early childhood* [II]. In : *The psychoanalytic study of the child*, **2**, 313
122. Stirnimann, F. (1933) *Das erste Erleben des Kindes*, Frauenfeld
123. Stumpfl, F. (1936) *Die Ursprünge des Verbrechens*, Leipzig
*124. Sutherland, E. H. (1947) *Principles of criminology*, 4th ed. Philadelphia
*125. Tappan, P. W. (1949) *Juvenile delinquency*, New York
126. Tramer, M. (1947) *Leitfaden der jugendrechtlichen Psychiatrie*, Basel
*127. Tramer, M. (1949) *Z. Kinderpsych.* **15**, 141
128. Tullio, B. di (1940) *Antropologia criminale*, Roma
129. United Nations, Economic and Social Council (1948) *Resolutions adopted by the Economic and Social Council during its seventh session from 19 July to 29 August 1948*, Geneva, resolution 155 (VII), page 33
130. United Nations, Economic and Social Council (1949) *Social Commission, fifth session. Report of the international group of experts on the prevention of crime and the treatment of offenders* (document E/CN.5/154)
131. Van Ophuijsen, J. H. W. (1945) *Primary conduct disturbances, their diagnosis and treatment, modern trends in child psychiatry*, New York
132. Vervaeck, L. (1939) *Syllabus du cours d'anthropologie criminelle*, Bruxelles
133. Wexberg, E. (1931) *Individualpsychologie*, Leipzig
134. White, R. W. (1948) *The abnormal personality*, New York
*135. *Why delinquency? The case for operational research : report of a conference on the scientific study of juvenile delinquency*, London, 1949 (containing particularly reports by Bowlby, J., Carroll, D., Mannheim, H., Pearce, J. D. W., Rodger, A. and Simey, T. S.)
136. Willcock, H. D. (1949) *Report on juvenile delinquency*, London
137. World Health Organization, Expert Committee on Mental Health (1950) *World Hlth Org. techn. Rep. Ser.* **9**
138. Yen, Ching-Yueh (1934) *Amer. J. Sociol.* **40**, 298
139. Young, P. V. (1930) *Publ. Amer. sociol. Soc.* **24**, 162
140. Young, P. V. (1932) *The pilgrims of Russian Town*, Chicago